# CELTIC REIKI
## STORIES FROM THE SACRED GROVE

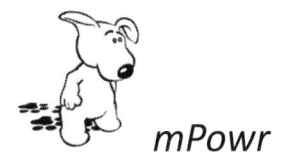

BY

## MARTYN PENTECOST

*mPowr*

© 2009 Martyn Pentecost

First Published in Great Britain 2009 by

mPowr (Publishing) Ltd.
Suite 11352, 2nd Floor, 145-157 St John Street, London EC1V 4PY

www.mpowrpublishing.com
www.mpowrunlimited.com

The moral right of the author has been asserted.

All rights Reserved. No part of this publication may be reproduced, stored in a retrieval system, or transmitted, in any form or by any means without the prior written permission of the publisher, nor be circulated in any form of binding or cover other than that in which it is published and without similar condition being imposed on the subsequent purchaser.

A catalogue record for this book is available from the British Library

ISBN – 978-1-907282-01-0

Cover Design by Martyn Pentecost
mPowr Publishing Clumpy™ Logo by e-nimation.com

Clumpy™ and the Clumpy™ Logo are trademarks of mPowr Ltd.

***Made by Book Brownies!***

Books published by mPowr Publishing are made by Book Brownies. A Book Brownie is about so high, with little green boots, a potato-like face and big brown eyes. These helpful little creatures tenderly create every book with kindness, care and a little bit of magic! Before shipping, a Book Brownie will jump into the pages— usually at the most gripping chapter or a part that pays particular attention to food—and stay with that book, always. This means that every mPowr Publishing book comes with added enchantment (and occasional chocolate smudges!) so that you get a warm, fuzzy feeling of love with the turn of every page!

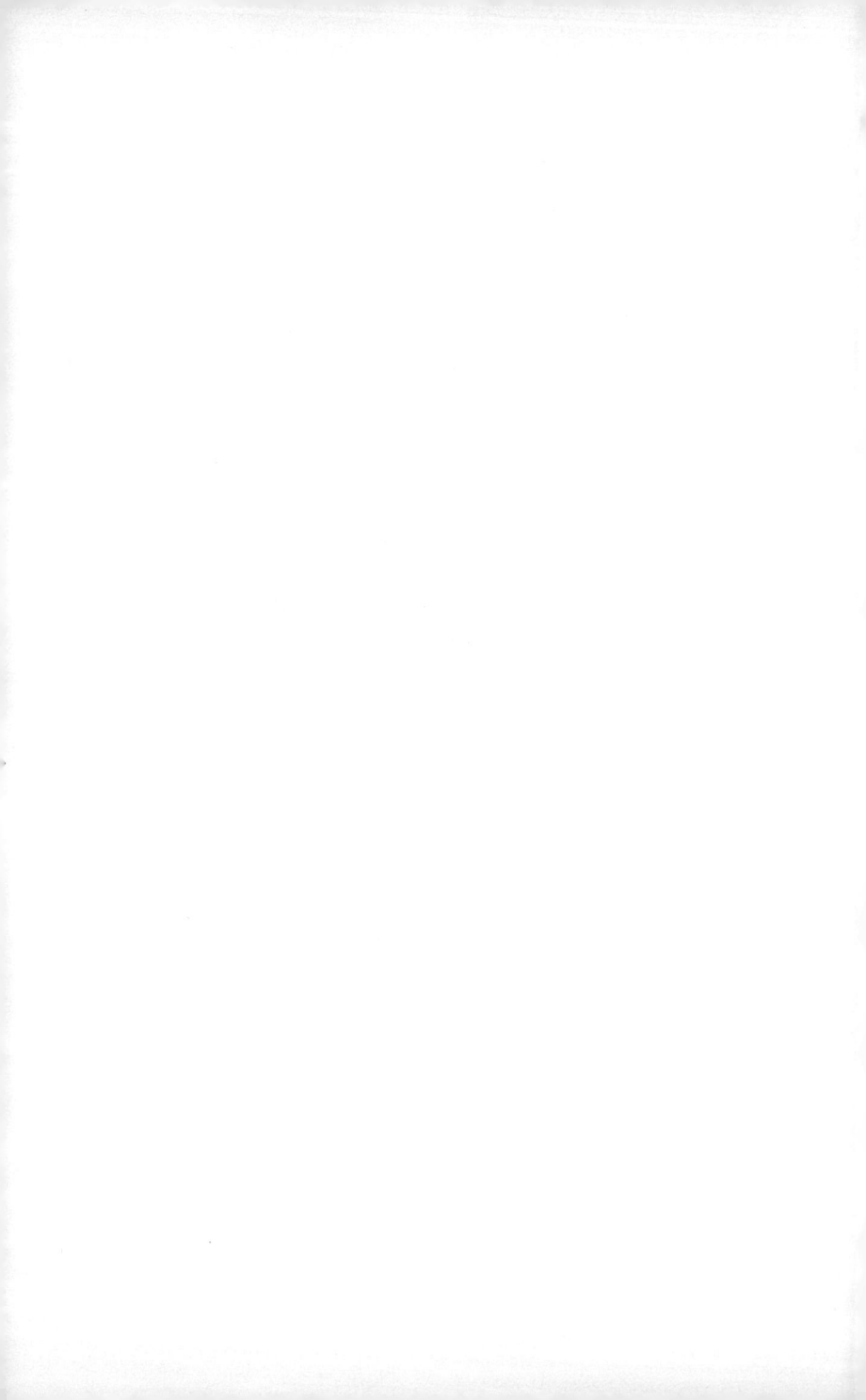

For the trees who helped to create this book...

...so that the wisdom and the beauty and the sacrifice of all their kind will not be forgotten.

# Contents

| | |
|---|---|
| A Journey Begins... | 9 |
| The Lost Language of Trees | 13 |
| Into the Forest | 19 |
| The Lone Tree | 23 |
| Yew Are Next! | 31 |
| A World of Enchantment | 39 |
| Making An Ash Of It... | 45 |
| Two Maples and a Blackbird | 53 |
| I Got The Ki, I Got The Secret! | 63 |
| Come Away, O Human Child! | 79 |
| The Little Christmas Tree | 89 |
| The Nameless Tree | 97 |
| The Psychic Years | 109 |
| A Lord of Thorns | 125 |
| Trouble and Straif | 131 |
| A Prickly Pair | 141 |
| It's Elemental, My Dear Watson! | 147 |
| The Bush That Burned | 155 |
| Farewell to Old Friends | 161 |
| The Essences of Celtic Reiki | 169 |
| Acknowledgements | 229 |

# A Journey Begins…

This is the story of Celtic Reiki. However it is not really a story in itself; it is more an invitation to a friend—an invitation to talk a while, to stroll on a beautiful day, listening to the birdsong and taking immense pleasure in feeling the sun on our faces. You see, for me the act of relating how Celtic Reiki came to be is not a cold undertaking of staring at a blank sheet as it fills with words: it is an interaction, it is a connection on a level that transcends words, it is a meeting in potential of two people who have a vast array of experiences to share.

From my perspective we know each other and we are simply reacquainting ourselves with some rather important information: we are all connected, we share this amazing world and we are all of the Earth. Let me explain by using an example that helped one of my students understand the world as I view it.

One day, Grandmother Sun gazed out at her children and saw that Father Earth was sad. She reflected for a moment and then asked, "Why are you so sad?"

"Because," Earth replied, "This morning I was born and everything felt cold. I was alone. Then I learnt to fly like an eagle across oceans and forests and mountains. I was free and I was alive."

"Sounds beautiful" Grandmother Sun murmured with introspection.

"But I was, in spite of everything, alone and up so high it was still cold. However, I then spied a community of rabbits, feasting and playing in a field. So I swooped down and became a rabbit. I lived and I loved. For many months I played in the field, I ate the lush grass and scented flowers. I fell in love and had children of my own."

Sensing that Father Earth had become quiet, the Sun offered encouragement. "Go on," she said.

"And then a man came and he killed my children and my companion. I was alone again. And I have never felt such grief or cried so hard."

"What did you do then?" The Sun asked, benevolently.

"I wanted to know why! I could not understand why the man could do this, why he needed to take away what I loved the most, why he needed to destroy! So, I became a man and then I discovered something that changed me so irrevocably that I will never be the same again!"

"As I stepped into the world as a man, I discovered how to express my joy, my freedom, my loneliness and pain in art, songs and books. I shared my grief and my love with others with each flicker of the screen and turn of the page. I learned how to connect with people in communities and societies, as friends and lovers. I feasted and made love. I saw the most beautiful skies, filled with stars. I made money and gained notoriety, I built cities and lived amongst many, just like in my rabbit warren. I flew in planes across oceans and forests, as if I were an eagle again."

"It sounds magical, my child" Grandmother Sun replied, respectfully. "And what did you learn?"

"In all my experiences, my memories and my dreams, I learnt that the world is a complex place, filled with love and hate, joy and pain. It is out of control and no matter what we do, it happens to us, we become involved in it and lost to it. No matter how free the eagle feels, she is still soaring alone, no matter how much the rabbit feels connection to his companions; that connection can be taken away. Regardless of the ability of a person to love, she can still choose to hate and does, even when those she hates never asked for, or needed, or deserved her hatred."

"And what did you forget?" Asked the Sun with a tone of knowing in her voice.

"Forget?" Replied the Earth. "I don't know!"

"You forgot that you are the Earth."

The Earth remained silent for a while.

"You are the Earth and every living thing that creates the Earth. You forgot that the eagle and the rabbit and the man are not separate from you. They are born of you. They are you and you are them! At any moment you are tasting the lush grass, or finding joy in the lyrics of a song. You are flying over oceans and gazing at the stars!"

"But it doesn't feel like that!" The Earth said suddenly.

"Of course not! When you are the Earth as a man, you act like a man and when you are the Earth as an eagle you fly like an eagle and when you are the Earth as a rabbit you feel like a rabbit—how else would you be able to commit to the moment and experience it as if it were real?"

"How do you know this?" The Earth whispered, quietly, yet urgently.

"Because I feel like a sun, I act like a sun, I shine. I give life and I take life away. I have been a sun for many millions of years and shall be millions more. However, this is not what I have always been and not what I will always be."

"What do you mean?" The Earth seemed puzzled.

"I am made of stardust. The molecules that create me were once stars in the ancient Universe, which were born, lived, and died in a blinding instant that appeared to be billions of years. You and I are both made of stardust and when we are gone, others will be born and live as who they are, but they will still be stardust. Every experience you have will be a part of that stardust, just as the memories of those long gone are part of you—if you just remember to listen."

# The Lost Language of Trees

It was just a little after daybreak on the idyllic shores of Loch Ness in Scotland. Winds from the mountains to the south were skimming the craggy slopes on the opposite bank before twisting on to the loch. As the fingers of this playful zephyr rippled the surface of the water, dark and mysterious shapes seemed to congregate below, reaching up to touch the air for a single, transitory moment. As the shadowy figures spread further across the loch, they seemed to reflect the ominous rain clouds that cascaded over the crest of the mountains.

    I was sitting on a rocky peninsula, listening to the low, rhythmic thud of the water as its foamy periphery clambered on to the rocks for an instant, before ebbing backwards into blackness. Warming sunlight on my face eased the morning chill in the damp air, the joyous chorus of songbirds saturated the air, and gradually I became completely enveloped by the power of this dynamic landscape. With each passing moment, I lost myself in this elaborate dance of life that existed all around me. This moment was all-encompassing, like the first bite of a sweet and juicy strawberry or the rapture of a favourite piece of music that elevates your soul to soaring new heights of pleasure.

I was brought back from my introspection by the invigorating breath of the wind that whispered portents of the approaching rain. The first few icy droplets on my cheek were in stark contrast to the vibrant heat of the sun and I felt as if I were sitting between worlds; the bright, sunlit, song-filled realm of the eastern forest and the dark, brooding mountains to the south.

For a while, I contemplated the thought of returning to the retreat house where I was facilitating an event that day. Yet, in awe of this beautiful place, I stayed. Knowing that this moment, right now, was precious, I decided that it was time to step outside of myself, to disconnect from the definitions of physical body and to connect to the observer; the 'I Am'. I realised, by my sitting at a point where the sun and rain met that I was in a very special place. So, I took my awareness to the mountainous slopes, towering above the loch and I gazed at the person perched on the rocks below. I watched, from afar, the man sitting at the end of the rainbow and I felt blissful in the knowledge that in everyday circumstances magic is everywhere, if only you look for it.

As I roused from my joyous state, I was aware of another presence; my happiness had caught the attention of a tiny oak sapling that was growing from the space between two boulders. This beautiful little being was only an arms-length from where I had been sitting, but he was so intent on remaining unnoticed that I had been unaware of his presence until then.

I reached out and held his delicate trunk in between my thumb and forefinger. He was thinner than a pencil, with his first leaves of spring just breaking from their buds. So young and frightened, this child, this living creature, knew so much of fear that I was saddened by the way he recoiled from my touch in terror.

"It's OK," I explained, in the Duir language of the Oak Tree, "I am here to listen and I want to help you."

The tree regarded me with bewilderment for a short while; a human who could speak the lost language of trees was indeed a curiosity. I just smiled and waited for him to gain enough confidence to reconnect with me. Then I asked him of his plans, his future, his wishes and dreams.

"Tell me," I enquired, "what are your plans for this coming year? What do you want to achieve?"

"To stay as small as I can" He replied timidly.

I was puzzled by his response and wanted to discover the reasons for his apathy. "You do not want to grow, to become tall and strong?"

He pondered this for a moment, before directing my attention to a place further along the shoreline, to where the three stumps of what were once the trunks of huge pine trees jutted from the rocks. This stark, cruel image and the pain of the little oak associated with it, were haunting. I glanced from this trio of fallen trees to the house where I was staying. I stared at the bay windows that offered such a beautiful view of the loch and I realised why these lives had been snuffed out.

"If I grow," said the oak, "they will cut me down."

It is not fitting of an oak tree to be afraid; I have only ever known them as noble, heroic, fearless and even though I have met individuals that could be deemed austere, they never display the slightest hint of trepidation. I held back the grief that erupted within me at the misguided logic of my species as the oak said in a whisper, "I don't want to die."

"I will tell you what to do," I explained with resolve. "You must strive every single moment of every day to be the best that you can be. Drink voraciously from the water of the loch, send your roots deeply into the ground, be flexible and bend with the wind, so that you grow up stronger and more beautiful than any other creature that lives in this place."

The oak remained silent for a while; this human was indeed peculiar!

"When you are the most wondrous sight on the shore of this place," I continued, "when you stand resilient and confident and powerful, when you fear nothing, you will not spoil their view of the loch; you will become their view of the loch. If you do this, they will never cut you down, because to do so, would ruin what they treasure most."

The oak took a while to reflect upon the notions of this unusual human, who not only spoke his language, but seemed to care deeply for his kind. As is the way with most trees, they do not rush or act quickly. Trees have more time than we can comprehend, so why miss the joy of a single moment by rushing to get there without enjoying the journey? Even baby trees take time to contemplate every challenge in relation to their perspective of the world; if they did not, they may miss out on the ecstasy each challenge brings!

Then I felt a rush of renewed courage burst from the tree as it made the decision to take my advice and with that overwhelming explosion came images of a long and glorious life, filled with happiness. As the sapling took his first step to being all that he could be, he chose a future where each and every second is relished, all seasons are experienced to the absolute full, and a lifetime is lived with nobility and serenity.

This little oak tree had determined with a single thought to squeeze every last drop of joy from a life that would span centuries. And I understood that in a brief, solitary flash of time I had guided this tree to a place where, no matter what happened in the future, he would achieve his dreams every single day.

It is the nature of our tree friends that when we offer them a gift, whether it be a drink of water on a hot day, a nourishing sprinkle of fertilizer when the ground is lacking, the planting of their seed, words of love, or actions that defend them when they cannot look after themselves, they offer a kindness in return. This tiny oak was no exception. He asked what he could do for me in return for taking the time to help him.

My answer was simple. I wanted him to remember. Remember the bright, spring morning when a man came and sat at the end of the rainbow. Remember this man who told him to be the best that he could be. To take a moment each day and remember. That way I could live in this magnificent place for many, many years to come and I would always be thought of with kindness and love.

As I said farewell to this most insignificant and profound of beings, I thought to myself how beautiful and perfect this morning had been. I reflected on how the choice to get every last drop of joy from my own life meant instilling this ideal in others. To know only love, bliss, and wonder, one must *be* love, bliss and wonder. It was at this moment that I made the decision to write this book as a way of sharing with you the discovery of how you too can be the best you can be. I wanted to share the moments I have experienced, in the hope that you may be inspired to find your bliss, your perfection. I offer you the insights that I discovered along the way.

So...when you are ready, pull up a rock, sit yourself down and know that you are at the end of the rainbow with somebody who has secrets to tell you. These secrets will lead you to places, sensations, emotions, and knowledge that are beyond your wildest imaginings. You will explore realms of infinite possibilities, learn to perceive the world in a very different way, and meet beings that love you with such an intense compassion that you never believed it was possible to be that adored.

On our journey together, we shall walk through woodlands, swim in the oceans, fly through the sky and travel where few people have ever gone before. And whilst you may be sitting on your rock, thinking that I'm talking to somebody else, one of the other people who are reading these words, you will come to realise that everything I show you is just for you...only you! How is this possible? Well, sit with me a while and I will show you how the world you thought you knew is actually an illusion—the truth is far more spectacular and beautiful...

# Into the Forest

Every tree in the forest has their own perspective, each species its own language and perception of the world in which they live. As a tree resonates into the environment in which it resides, the neighbouring trees comprehend this resonance from a partially contrasting viewpoint; they translate their companion's resonance with slightly different translations and beliefs. This means that each surrounding tree takes from the resonance its own personal message that changes and evolves with time. The lost language of the trees is never static or stagnant: it is constantly fluid and changing, adapting to the circumstances and needs of the moment.

   This language has become severely atrophied since it was commonly used as an integral part of the Celtic culture in Western Europe. Our modern day society has all but forgotten what it is to be a part of the natural world; to exist in balance and harmony with the trees and the wildlife that create the complex ecosystems of our world. Trees are mostly viewed as a commodity, whilst animals are classed as expendable by many. We value human life above all else and in many ways, this is part of our very necessary survival instinct. However, it is my belief that our ability to take from the world is the very ability that enables us act as custodians of this planet and our precious natural realms.

Our intelligence is remarkable—we are remarkable—wonderful beings that walk in the physical world and dance in the light. We need to eat, to drink, to breathe so that our bodies; our anchors into this solid world can carry us. Yet, we tend not to use what we need in a balanced way, we take to excess. We have allowed our Western society to focus us solely on the physical and have turned away from our vibrant, energy selves. Nevertheless, this is changing. As more and more people undergo a reawakening to their light, their power, their potential, we are seeing a global shift, back to the old traditions and forward to our advanced future selves, who can implement those traditions without the often brutal practices that necessitated them.

My own journey has taken me across continents and through many contrasting cultural traditions. It has spanned many years and encompassed infinite realms of wisdom. The rediscovery of a non-human language, which has been almost completely forgotten, the creation of healing therapies that have captured the imagination of thousands of people, and the expansion of perception to encompass many thousands of years into the past and future are all a part of this journey.

And as you walk with me a while, we will share the understanding that I cannot tell you what you 'have to do' to achieve this for yourself; because my truth is not your truth. Instead, you can experience the knowledge I have gained along the way, the interactions with some very special individuals, and the philosophies of those that exist beyond our everyday perception. We will traverse psychology, linguistics, psychic abilities, healing, spirituality, sexuality, and emotional wellbeing, along with an infinite realm of other topics of conversation...with this, you will have enough information to discover your own unique perspective of your life and the world around you.

This is the discovery of your own truth—a truth that has not been dictated to you and forced upon you, but that you have nurtured and developed all by yourself. Just as the resonant tree offers a message that is Universal, the surrounding trees give that resonance meaning from their own unique viewpoint. Here is my message, my journey—in it you will see the parallels in your own life and, hopefully, you will connect to your own inner guidance through those parallels.

# The Lone Tree

It was a dark and rainy autumnal day when I made the very first step towards the creation of the self-development system, now known as Celtic Reiki. I was visiting a small village on the border of Wales and Shropshire, slowly meandering around the local cemetery. I enjoyed the sensation of the cool rain on my face, as I weaved my way amongst the ancient headstones, occasionally stopping to read the epitaphs and consider the lives of those who died so long ago.

It makes me smile that almost everybody I have met in my psychic work says cemeteries are not in the least bit frightening; in fact they are incredibly restful places. I agree entirely! As a child I would visit Hampstead Cemetery in London with my Grandmother on a regular basis. Each week I would help her tend the graves of our relatives; I would often ask questions about death and what was to come after we died, she would say that those we love watch over us, which explained why the lady in a white nightgown was always looking at me from the grave of my Great Aunt.

After my Grandmothers death, I spent many hours weeping in that same cemetery, under the sheltering branches of a weeping willow tree who seemed to understand my grief and hid me from the passers-by, who could not see through the thick curtain of leaves. Hence, I feel it was a fitting gesture that this same willow would later become the 'Weeping Tree of Sanctuary' in the Celtic Reiki system.

It is a comfort to me that Celtic Reiki was born in such a peaceful and beautiful place as that little Welsh cemetery: a place that shared the same atmosphere as so many of my fondest childhood memories, where the dead watch over us as the living heal their grief and sorrow. This amazing balance of life, death and rebirth was so revered by the Celts that it imbued their perspective of our tree friends. The old, the new, the past, the future and the now, the cycles of the seasons and of all living things were mirrored in that first meeting I had with the Lone Tree.

This magnificent Fir tree stood alone at the west face of the cemetery chapel and it dominated the view, being the tallest tree in the locale. There was a majesty and quiet air of austerity about this beautiful creature that made the scene even more devastating. At first I was shocked at the sheer scale of the destruction, this was not simply an act of nature—it seemed violent, almost hostile in appearance.

The fir had been struck by lightning and cloven completely into two pieces: one still standing, the other lying a few feet away. Shattered pieces of wood and bark were scattered all around as a testament to the ferocious nature of the storm that resulted in this, almost awe-inspiring scene. The restless, brooding sky darkened over the twisted wreckage of the tree's once sturdy trunk, threatening in the small droplets of rain to continue its onslaught.

I felt absolutely compelled to do something that would, in some way, alleviate what I perceived as the tree's pain. Looking back, I know that I have witnessed many fallen trees before and after the Lone Tree event and none have affected me as profoundly or as deeply as this one incidence. The cycle of life and death in the forest is a natural flow, which the trees accept and are an integral, willing participant in. This scene appeared so cruel and vehement in its destruction that I was totally overwhelmed by what I can only describe as despair.

The images of that day hold close connections for me to an earlier memory from my 'scientifically orientated' twenties. I was looking after a friend's cat when she started to die in front of me. Her death was so unexpected and sudden that all ability to think simply went. I sat, a weeping mess on the floor holding her in my arms, wishing that I could believe in some 'other place', where 'some benevolent force' would look after her and keep her safe. I desperately wanted to have faith in the idea that she was now playing with butterflies in flower-filled, sunlit fields, but my scientifically sceptical atheism prevented me from understanding anything other than the lights going out and an endless, dreamless sleep.

This was the day I realised that despite all the questions my scientific training had answered, there was one question that it could not answer. For all the practical uses for science in our world, none of the disciplines I had invested so much of my time in could offer me hope or help me to save this life that ebbed into nothingness against my chest. That was the day I decided I needed to find a different philosophy; one that could provide me with something more than our solid, material existence.

Soon after I started to explore the concepts of Metaphysics and Transpersonal Psychology, which led me to the energy therapy known as Usui Reiki. It was through my Reiki Mastership training that I discovered the answers to those questions that had evaded me for so long and it was Reiki that enabled me to believe in something more when I happened upon the Lone Tree in the little village cemetery.

As I walked towards the tree, my hands started to tingle with heat that expanded outwards with a radiance that could best be described as 'fierce'. This was a sure sign that the Reiki had activated and I was ready to do some form of treatment for the tree. At that point, I was unsure about what I could do to help, but the need to take some form of action was overwhelming. So, as I neared the tree, I started by placing my hands around the shattered trunk and clearing my mind.

Something was not right, the connection to Reiki started to wane and I felt as if the tree was not comfortable with the treatment, or that it was refusing my help in some way. I gazed down at the mangled remains of the fallen half of Fir tree and wondered if treating this part of the tree might be a better use of time. Thus, reaching through the thick, needle-filled branches, I placed my hands on the bare wood and attempted to increase my Reiki connection.

Again this was to no avail. I could certainly feel the life ebbing away from the tangled remains, yet all the usual sensations of the Reiki connection just were not there. So I stepped back for a moment and considered the situation. The answer came in a flash of inspiration, which in retrospect seems so obvious, however at the time I just was not accustomed to working with trees! Thus I crouched down and reached out, once again, through the needle-covered branches of the dying part of the Fir, although this time I only used my left hand. With the right arm, I lifted my hand and placed it on the wound of the upright section. My intent was to create some form of bridge between the living and the dying; a link that would enable the gradually diminishing life to reconnect with the part of the tree that was still standing.

I was overwhelmed by the sudden jolt of vibrancy that felt as though it were clambering up the inside of my left arm. Concurrently, the right arm became alive with a contrasting sensation; similar to the Reiki connection I was familiar to, yet somehow different. These two vibrant feelings converged in the heart and head areas of my body and at once, I was wrapped in the most indescribable joy. When I reminisce about the moments in my life where I have touched the Divine, this is one of those clearest and most profound. The benevolence, compassion and sheer yearning to experience every wonderful drop of life created a fleeting glimpse of perfection.

My whole body juddered as the vibrations clambered to an astonishing crescendo of sensation, emotion and expansion. I experienced a voice; not the sound of a voice that we would be accustomed to in the physical world, but more like a version of my own internal monologue. This voice however was very deep and resonant; it boomed through me, like the reverberation of thunder, or the pounding of violent ocean waves, crashing against the shore. I cannot describe the effect as sound, for even the loudest of sounds was not like this. It did not originate from the external world, it was a part of me; as if every cell of my body resounded with the message in unison.

The voice echoed the words "Thank you", and, "this will help people to see." The second of these seemed cryptic at first, nevertheless I continued to crouch and sizzle away with energy, until a further shift slipped me into the familiar Reiki connection.

As I completed the treatment by returning both hands to the standing tree, I felt a wholeness that had not existed before. Glancing down at the torn remains I could see there was nothing left except for the wood. At the time, it appeared as though the 'life-force' of the tree had passed through me from the dying limbs to the surviving section of the tree, thus the cloven Fir had been made whole once again. Over the years, my attitude to this incident has evolved somewhat and I now believe that I initiated a connection, not only between the two halves of the tree, but also within myself and within the Universe. This coming together of the shattered and the ripped-apart was the catalyst that not only sparked the healing of the Fir tree; it also started a deep healing process within me. In addition to my own healing journey, I have noticed along the way how the world seemed different after that day, as a result of my interaction with the Fir. The world did not change for the better—my perspective of the world changed for the better!

Latterly, I have used a similar connection technique to help trees that are dying in finding a new life; on some occasions carrying a connection around with me whilst searching for a suitable anchor for the vibrational force. The technique can be found exclusively in the *Celtic Reiki Workbook*.

As the Reiki treatment drew to a close, I thanked the Fir tree for letting me help and for offering such a wonderful experience in return! As I walked away, I knew I was changed, internally and irrevocably. What I had yet to realise was just how that single incident would change my life and become the first chapter in a personal-development modality that would spread across the globe.

Soon after the Lone Tree connection, I started to notice a very similar 'internal monologue' experience to that which I had whilst 'bridging' the two halves of the tree. On these subsequent occasions, however, the voices altered from experience to experience. As I encountered trees on the street or whilst walking in the countryside, they would offer arbitrary pieces of information, such as how they were 'feeling', or what the weather would be doing next week! Sometimes they would give advice, express an opinion, or assist me in some other way. This initially disconcerting development triggered within me a need to know more. So I started to research traditional beliefs surrounding trees.

It was during my research that I came across the Celtic philosophies and principles, and it was from these basic foundations that I discovered the Fir Tree was associated with the ability to see into the future. This intuitive ability is derived from the Fir Tree's height and therefore, its ability to 'see' much further than other trees. In the modern writings, the Fir is often referred to as Ailim (Arl-m), which also has connections to the Elm Tree. This was how the first Essence in Celtic Reiki happened to be the first letter in the Celtic Ogham or alphabet.

# Yew Are Next!

Over the next few months, I slipped into a realm of enchantment that seemed different from the everyday world. This is, in so many ways, a real challenge to put into words, because words simply do not portray the utterly core-wrenching nature of such a vivid, all-encompassing experience. Nonetheless, let me start with the colour green, which may seem a rather unusual place to begin in connection to the term 'core-wrenching', yet it is rather fitting, as you will see.

    I have always loved colour. In fact, one of my party pieces as a very young child was to describe the colours of passing car. This activity always astonished my mother, as I did not simply suggest the colours of red, blue, green and so on, I was a little more descriptive. 'Puce' is not really the sort of expression a parent is used to hearing their two-year-old articulate, unless of course they are mispronouncing another activity that we won't go into. Coral, azure, ochre, ultramarine, olive, or vermillion are also not usually a part of a pre-schooler vocabulary, although I would happily recite these correctly from my pushchair.

    Now at this juncture, you are almost certainly asking one of two questions; the first being, how did I know these words and their associated colours? The second is why were there ochre and coral coloured cars on the street? The latter is an easy query to answer; it was the Seventies! The initial question is a slightly greater challenge, because I simply do not know where I learnt to name those colours so accurately. The knowledge was just 'there'.

Thinking back, colours and their descriptive names were some of the first things I can remember knowing. They were so integral to my being that I would spend hours creating colour coded lists or painting pictures using elaborate shading and minute transitions of colour. I was so focussed on colour that I can recall pestering my mother, one birthday, to bake a cake with chartreuse tinted icing on top. I did not care about anything other than that precise colour of decoration. That was the year I learnt that 'chartreuse' is grown-up code for 'the shade of baby poo'. After that, I did not ask my mum to bake me a cake with any form of ornamentation, chromatic or otherwise!

As I grew older, my eyesight became my weaker and I started to lose definition on the edges of objects. This meant that I relied even more on colours to conceptualise the world I saw around me. In fact, much of my adult life has been, visually, a kaleidoscope of coloured blurs, because rather than distinct forms or shapes, I see the world in tiny differences in shade, tone and luminosity. I can spot minute differences in pantone colouration, though ask me to read a car registration at 50 feet and I would be more likely to come runner-up in a gurning competition than actually get the correct answer!

It was because of having such a defined acuity in the visual sense that after the interaction with the cloven Fir tree, I found the colour green overwhelming. For it was as though somebody had suddenly turned up the colour saturation on the green! From the vibrant lime green of beech tree leaves, to the emerald green of grass, everywhere I looked, the entire green spectrum was more dazzling than ever.

Furthermore, all plants appeared to take on a bizarre luminosity, similar to that of the auric field, which surrounds all living things and yet, different. It was as though this pale, electric-blue light was burnt into my vision, like the after-effects of staring at a bright light and the imprint that is temporarily left behind. What made this all the more remarkable was that it appeared to give definition to the finer details of the plants. For the first time I could see branches, buds, leaves, leaf veins and the ripples of bark in the most exquisitely refined detail. Yet these were not the sharp lines of perfect vision; it was what I can best describe as the sight of an 'inner-knowing' or seeing the life-force of the plant, as opposed to the visual definition of its body.

An even more baffling visual effect was soon to become apparent, as I started to see shapes amongst groups of trees or, on some occasions, connected to a single tree. These elongated or oval patches of hazy light gave the impression of floating about a foot off the ground and would sometimes by moving slowly, sometimes completely still. These shapes were not merely flat distortions; they would change in shape as I moved around them, akin to how a three-dimensional object alters with a modification in perspective.

If I slipped my hand into the space occupied by these shapes, they would buzz and tingle, similar to an effervescent drink fizzing away on my skin. The most disquieting aspect of these shapes was a very tangible feeling of being watched. I soon came to believe that these were sentient entities; as aware of my presence as I was of theirs, and actually responsive to it.

Were these the really the mythical dryads or tree spirits the Celts revered and worshipped? Perhaps I had actually come to sense fairy-folk? Whatever they were, as time went on and I worked with an ever-increasing number of trees, my sensory information about these creatures became significantly refined.

It was soon after my connection to the Lone Tree that I visited the small town of Painswick in Gloustershire, UK. This deliciously quaint place is the site of the 99 Yew Trees, which stand, perfectly manicured, in St. Mary's Churchyard. According to local folklore, if ever a hundredth tree is planted in the grounds, the Devil will pluck it out.

I do not know whether the Devil has an interest in Yew trees or not, however, I have spent a lot of time over the years immersed in the amazing ambience of the churchyard. It was these striking trees that first formed the Essence of Ioho; the Yew Essence. One tree in particular guided me through this process and when I say 'guided', it is testament to the level of enchantment I was beginning to feel at the time.

The Yew tree that I primarily worked with in the churchyard of St Mary's first grabbed my attention as an 'internal monologue' that after the Lone Tree had become increasingly apparent. Whenever I was in the proximity of the tree, my thoughts would turn to endings, to the cycle of life and death, and what happens to us when we embark on that great unknown voyage at the end of our lives. A single phrase would turnaround in my head, it seemed to be telling me that the tree would "guide me beyond endings".

After many passes of the tree, I finally decided to stand next to him and listen for a while. Gradually I was prompted to place my hands around his trunk and create a connection. This was the first time that I performed the technique that is now known in therapies such as Celtic Reiki and Lemuria as 'Harvesting'.

Now, I don't know if you have ever hugged a tree in public, but the first time can be quite disconcerting, especially at three in the afternoon with camera-wielding tourists and a fair few locals milling about. In retrospect, any town that is used to the Devil stalking its Yew trees with malicious intent, would pay little attention to a strange, tree-hugging Londoner. However, I did not think that way in the inaugural months of Celtic Reiki creation. Now, of course, I flit from tree to tree like an oversized wood-nymph, hugging trees with a voracity that is more floozy-like than nymph-like!

So, now that I've put that colourful image in your head, let me tell you one of the most valuable lessons I was taught by that first Yew tree. I stood, experiencing his vibrations and listening to a voice that seemed so young on one level, yet ancient in the wisdom it imparted. In a semi-trance-like state, I found myself wondering what the Yew tree energy 'did'; as in, what it could be used for therapeutically. The tree slowed for a moment and commented upon my introspection.

"Don't ask what a tree can do for you." He whispered, gently, "ask the tree what you can do for him."

I gleaned two lessons here. The first being that if you want to keep secrets from trees, don't think about those secrets when you are in the middle of a hug—they will comment on them (and some can be rather less than diplomatic!) Secondly and more importantly, this: we ask so much of our tree friends, whether it be using them for wood or chopping them down, because they 'spoil' our view. Most people do not even spare a thought for trees, let alone other plant-life, ripping it from the ground without a second thought or word of apology. There are very few tears shed over trees that die of sickness or are uprooted by the wind. Even fewer for the trees whose lives we snuff out. The one bastion of dignity they have is their energy, their spirit. We cannot take that from them and if we want to share their essence, by immersing ourselves in it physically, emotionally, mentally and spiritually, the least we can do is to share something of ourselves (though perhaps not the aforementioned secrets!)

It was at that moment I began to cultivate the most vital habit when connecting to trees. I asked, "What can I offer you?"

"Tell me about your fears," the tree replied.

It was at this point that I wondered if all that 'living in fear of a jolly good Devil-uprooting' had turned the tree into a bit of a fear-junkie, but nevertheless, I started to reflect on my own fears. And as I thought about them, they left me. I searched deeper and deeper into my past and my subconscious mind to try and ease out any buried fears that I could relate to the tree, but as I found a fear, it seemed to dissipate under my conscious focus.

I soon realised that it was the Yew who was releasing my fear and that it was not a case of him wanting to know my fears; it was that me asking what he wanted from me was enough of a kindness for him to reciprocate. You see trees are custodians. They were here long before any creature walked on the Earth, or flew across the sky. They give us air to breathe and make it possible for us to live, so in many ways, they are like parents to us all.

Now some trees are deeply suspicious of humankind and can be quite austere (catch an Oak tree on a bad day and your hands will sting for a week!) However, like most parents, they forgive and if you show them kindness, they offer in return a benevolence and love that is beyond anything you can imagine. It is what I can best describe as the Earth itself loving you.

The early tribal communities lived in complete harmony with the Earth. They knew everything exists in balance and, to survive, they needed to be in harmony with the rest of the world.

As *modern* humans 'evolved', we started to adapt the environment around our own needs and desires. So we fell out of sync with the world, losing what it is to be a part of the amazingly intricate plan. We discovered loneliness and isolation. To compensate we became even more fixated on material gain and the adaptation of the outside world: creating cities; big businesses, and acquiring an unremitting need for personal possessions. When we discover a way of returning to equilibrium, through the practices of Celtic Reiki for instance, the feelings and sensations are literally awe-inspiring. Things become simpler and we reclaim the deep-rooted knowledge that we are totally loved. In other words, we simply become enchanted.

# A World of Enchantment

An interesting fact about originating an energy therapy that I can state from experience is how many mistakes there are to be made. Actually, I now regard these as opportunities to mature, whilst bringing something of even greater value into the world. If Celtic Reiki had coalesced perfectly, without the occasional dead-end or wrong direction, it would have been a very different (and I do feel, not as 'sincere') system.

I've lived with Celtic Reiki for about a third of my life; I've grown up with it and with each assumption that needed to be re-examined or misjudged each action that led to frustration, I have grown up a little more. Sometimes I've learnt quickly, as in following my intuition with the treatment of the Lone Tree, or by appreciating the prerequisite of reciprocation with the Painswick Yew.

There are, however, also times when my education was painfully slow. For example, it took a number of years before I understood that we cannot simply impose our will on trees in the hope of getting something from them; their Essence needs to be earned. Some trees will give their Essence freely or without much need for reciprocation, conversely there are those individuals that may take months of work and gesture before allowing a harvesting to take place (we shall visit the Sanctuary Oak later!)

A wonderful aspect of Celtic Reiki is that it is incredibly forgiving of one's rather excessive need to mature and all the opportunities that requires! As I practised with the Fir and the Yew elements of this exhilarating new therapy I was creating, I wholeheartedly threw myself into the creation of something much more elaborate. Studying the Celtic traditions and in particular the Ogham, I assigned the letter 'A' to the Fir Essence (Ailim) and 'I' to the Yew (Ioho). I also noted how similar my experiences of the Essences in treatment were to the beliefs of the Celtic peoples.

With such a huge array of choices to be made and paths to walk down, I was led by modern writings on the Celtic traditions. Identifying some of the sacred trees in the 'Celtic perspective', I acquired several Essences, by offering Reiki to trees and then harvesting the 'echo' or vibrations that resounded back.

With a system of around eighteen Essences, I rigorously tested each layer of Celtic Reiki, relishing all the feedback and honing the effectiveness of the treatments. The results were astounding, with my clients responding much more to Celtic Reiki than the other treatment modalities I used. So, after an extensive period of creation, I developed a style of teaching, based on the Usui Reiki 'attunement' processes, and began to teach Celtic Reiki to others.

Celtic Reiki spread around the world very quickly. People seemed to discover a deep resonance with the tree Essences and the 'Earth-centred' ethos behind the practice. I received letters and emails from people as far apart as Australia and South America. The United States and Canada became massive centres for Celtic Reiki practice and the course materials for teaching the values and principles were translated into various European languages.

I was stunned by the popularity of the therapy at first, not quite comprehending why a practice that was based upon the synergistic combination of ancient Western European and Japanese traditions would turn out to be so compelling across contrasting cultures and languages. I now realise, of course, that it is not the perspective of Celtic Reiki that created such a connection for people; it is the compassion of the trees and the engrained wisdom of the Earth that those who touch Celtic Reiki become so intrinsically linked with.

I watched as my little child went out into the world and grew up with guardians from every way of life, status and attitude. Eventually, I moved on to the development of other therapies, such as Ascension Energy Therapy (AET), Karmic Reiki (now Karmic Regression Therapy) and Lemuria.

In 2004, however, Celtic Reiki came back to me and since that time, it has been a regular companion. With the addition of many new Essences, including non-Celtic trees and 'elemental' Essences, such as Water (Dwr) and Fire (Tan), Celtic Reiki now possesses a vast range of treatment methodologies and a very different philosophy to those early days. What is more, the use of Celtic Reiki has benefited more people than I could ever have imagined and it is the stories from those whose lives have changed as a result of Celtic Reiki that move me the most.

Stories have actually become an integral part of Celtic Reiki practice; the art of allegory, fable and metaphor help us to grasp new ideas or ancient wisdom that may be alien to our current perspective. For example, the concept of Ki, and how the various facets of Ki interweave into a perfectly balanced dynamic, was quite a lot to get my head around at first; it was through analogy that I discovered how to comprehend the different cultural viewpoint of Ki. Considering that Ki had been repackaged and homogenised for the Western mindset, revisiting the foundations of Ki and, in particular Reiki philosophy, revolutionised my Reiki practice and my world view. It did take a while to filter through my existing 'schema' and alter the way I perceive everything.

Now this ancient tradition is part of who I am and I understand the principles of Ki in a very tangible and complex way. I would never have reached that level of complexity if it were not for the transmission of stories. In the same way as a ball and a dog can help a child to learn the intricacies of the English language, fantastical tales can convey ideas and thoughts that on their own would simply bounce off our conscious filters into oblivion!

Just as the Celts used parables to hand down spiritual knowledge from generation to generation, the transfer of wisdom in Celtic Reiki reflects this same ritual. Not only because it is such a fun way to learn, but also because it brings us closer to how the trees communicate and how the force of Ki is transmitted from living thing to living thing. By emulating the energy of trees and Ki, we not only learn how Celtic Reiki works, we are acting in exactly the same manner as the source elements.

Hence, as Ki transforms into different facets for different purposes and trees share their own perspective to attain a better understanding of the world beyond their own perception. Stories give us these same abilities; we change and evolve through emulation of the processes of adaptation and shared communication. Stories touch us deeply emotionally and psychologically, plus we can adapt those same stories to encompass the changes they created within us. As stories alter us, we alter them; forming a fluid way of teaching and learning.

Of course, this was one of those lessons that did not come easily. In fact it was a rather embarrassing and potentially humiliating incident that taught me the value of stories and the importance of flexibility in their telling.

# Making An Ash Of It...

One of the most valuable (and at the time embarrassing) lessons for me whilst on my Celtic Reiki journey comes from the teachings of a most beautiful Ash tree in North London. I had been asked to participate in a television interview about trees with a well-known British comedian. I arrived, with some trepidation, to discover that the funny anecdotes I had carefully prepared beforehand were not quite what the producers had in mind; I was to be introduced as one of the 'tree experts', along with the renowned Botanist, David Bellamy.

Now I have had many close encounters of the 'televisual' kind and there are two that stand out in my memory as the most horrifically embarrassing moments anybody could ever wish for. And, quite coincidentally, both involved the aforementioned Mr Bellamy! The first was, as a ten-year-old, being asked to do a vocal impression of him on live television, which still gives me the chills and not in a good way. The second was being equated with the same degree of arboreal knowledge as him and then being questioned by a comedian with a reputation for making his interviewees come across as slightly peculiar—and believe me, I don't need any help in that department!

I have the clearest recollection of walking down a long gravel pathway on this beautiful summer day, heading towards the film crew and thinking, "They're going to ask me to hug trees and talk like David Bellamy!"

Now, in retrospect, this request should not have bothered me in the slightest, because I am actually rather partial to the occasional bit of tree-hugging. In fact, many a tree has commented that I have quite an accomplished technique when it comes to hugging! As for the talking like David Bellamy, well, it couldn't be any more of a traffic accident than the first time and this wasn't live so I had plenty of takes to perfect my craft!

It is of course rather fitting that the term 'traffic accident' be applied in relation to this particular episode of my Celtic Reiki adventures, because what was about to transpire was nothing short of a proverbial Juggernaut, hurtling towards my reputation as a (virtually) sane person. So, forgive me for repeating myself, but if they wanted peculiar...

Now, before I continue, let me just mention that, what was to be Celtic Reiki's one and only BBC extravaganza never, in reality, made it to people's screens. In fact, when they aired the show some months later, I made the decision not partake in the end result, as the thought of sitting, watching through clasped fingers was not something that filled me with a warm and fluffy glow. However a student of mine, who did watch it, described the programme as being nothing, but 'bums and chicken legs'. Ahem...obviously I wasn't quite in the loop of just how big a traffic accident they were expecting me to be. There are some things I just will not do for my art!

So there we were; a small band of intrepid explorers, preparing to delve into the unknown realms of bums, chicken legs and soon-to-be cut trees (this was possibly the only occasion when I agreed with trees being cut!) I was introduced to said comedian, who was lovely, very respectful and charming. A small microphone was wired to my person and we were ready. Everything was just right, the sunlight dappled through the leaves of the Ash tree, a gentle breeze teased the branches, and the only sounds were a soft rustle of the surrounding trees and the melodic songs of birds high above us. We were all eager to embark on this exploration of Celtic Reiki, so it was not long before the cameras starting rolling.

Neither was it long before the microphone died, the planes started flying over head with painfully loud constancy and the instantaneous hurricane-style winds blew in a mini-apocalypse. Despite all of these interruptions we eventually arrived at the first question..."So, tell me about Celtic Reiki?"

I started eloquently, relating the Japanese origins of Reiki and how trees were perceived as sacred by the Celtic people. This inspired the question, "Why were trees sacred?"

Another brief bout of audio-equipment malfunction, planes and mini-apocalypse gave me enough time to move beyond the "What makes anything sacred?" response I was about to volunteer and speak poetically about Celtic traditional beliefs surrounding the forest deities and the spiritual importance of trees. I would have spoken at greater length, poetically or otherwise, if I had known what was about to transpire, however the blissful nature of my unawareness led me tippy-toe-ing confidently into the realm of tree-induced, vehicular carnage! Let me just state that no trees or vehicles were harmed in the making of these memories, though one Celtic Reiki Master's ego was severely mangled!

As I came to the natural completion of my answer, there was a slight, almost imperceptible shift in the comedian's eyes as he switched from the role of interviewer and focussed on showing his wide-eyed TV audience a hilarious display of rampant tree-lovin'. This ever-so-slight change in outward appearance was accompanied with the question, "So what do you do actually do with the trees?"

"Oh, Celtic Reiki Masters harvest the Essences of trees and then use them to help other people heal or create wellbeing." I replied, innocently.

Sometimes my own naivety shocks me to my very core, because at the precise moment of saying those words, the voice in my head was screaming at me not to say those words. Yet, despite my inner-wisdom having an episode, I decided that everything was good; after all, this polite, courteous TV personality would not do anything to make me look ridiculous, would he!

The whole world in all its incomprehensible complexity and diversity seemed to decelerate to a virtual halt as the following words were formed from the presenter's lips and travelled across the air to my ears. "Can you demonstrate how you would do that?"

There was an odd silence that permeated my entire being and lingered for the longest moment, until the aforementioned 'inner-wisdom' produced some rather choice advice for me, which went something along the lines of... "You silly, silly Boy!"

This slow-mo reality (and the aftermath) are characteristic of so many of the moments we experience in Celtic Reiki Mastership; profound flashes of inexpressible wonder, when everything stops in a single instant of perfection. I can recall many, many instances in my own experience of Celtic Reiki that transcend time, space and everyday consciousness. Fragments of pure connection, when the whole world is utterly beautiful and the sense of being enveloped in an infinite, loving benevolence is felt to the very foundations of one's being.

This was not one of those moments. No, this was another type of slow-mo reality that was akin to the fraction of a second which is sandwiched between tripping over a random cat and smacking oneself, head-first on to parquet flooring. You know that fraction of a second, which lasts long enough for you to think thoughts such as, "What was that cat doing there?" "Why are cats so random?" and "My my, isn't that parquet flooring moving fast!"

"Of course I can!" I replied as the fragmented figments of parquet flooring jangled into the past. "We can work with this Ash Tree here!"

There was an air of expectancy surrounding the various people who watched as I moved to the trunk of the tree. The clean, crisp desire to produce compulsive television was about to be fulfilled as I stretched out my arms and placed my hands around the trunk of the ancient Ash. This was to be the last action I consciously controlled for the rest of the interview and whilst I sometimes wonder if most of my actions have any connection with the concept of conscious control, this was something unlike any experience before or since.

The effect of touching the tree was akin to placing one's head on an old washing machine, whilst on spin cycle. Actually, I should clarify that I have never in reality placed my head on an old washing machine, whilst on spin cycle (neither myself, nor the washing machine), the sensation was how I imagine that particular activity to feel like. The overwhelming vibration that flooded up my arms and into my head, achieved what I can best describe as a disconnection from conscious control. It was as if my internal monologue was divorced from the words, gestures and movements that became manifest from the body. Imagine sitting in some distant place above yourself, watching and listening as something too hideous for words plays out in front of you!

The comedian wrapped himself around the tree and after a brief interlude, explained with glee that he could not feel anything. To which I slurred some inane response, whilst wondering if something had happened to his nerve endings in the same way as something had happened to my sanity!

The descent into the realm of the verbally ineffective continued as I explained that trees were my best friend and laughed raucously at the veiled suggestion that I had a tree 'girlfriend' tucked away. This horrific display tumbled toward the finale with one last question...

"Why do you like trees so much?" There was a pause, in which the distance I experienced between my consciousness and the point of Juggernaut collision appeared to stretch out even further as I heard four little words come out of my mouth.

"They make great furniture!"

At that moment I seriously thought the comedian's eyes were going to pop out of his head. His jaw literally dropped and the silent gasp of bewilderment that was stifled from those watching could almost be heard. Suddenly, all those years of passionately defending our tree friends flooded through my mind. Years of pushing the boundaries of how people perceive the 'wooden things with leaves on', the heartbreak I have felt, watching humankind treat these precious living creatures as commodities to be chopped down and used without respect, the wonderment I have known when discovering the individual personality of another tree friend.

Suddenly my self-definition as a Tree Advocate melted into the vision of becoming a spokesperson for IKEA. People across the UK would witness my smiling face, accompanied with the words, "They make great furniture!" And Celtic Reiki Masters across the globe would have a new slogan for their publicity material "Come and be treated with Essence of small coffee table!"

I was appalled at myself and was just unable to understand what had gone so awry. As the interview concluded and I was left dazed from what had happened, the approaching voice of the director snapped me back into reality. To complete the interview, they wanted a thirty second interstitial of me standing by the tree and staring out into space—presumably in search of some semblance of coherent thought. So I clambered up the bank and rested against the lowest branches of the tree, standing vacantly, like some form of rationality-bereft French Lieutenant's Woman.

With my hands holding one of the tree's larger boughs, another of those slow-mo moments began. The instantly recognisable vibrations of Nuin (The Celtic Reiki Essence of the Ash tree) saturated my awareness, leaving me totally confused. The tree was laughing!

"Why?" I ask the playful Ash, "Why did this happen?"

The tree replied and with a sense of utter care and compassion, explained to me a piece of wisdom that changed my life forever. This wisdom did not come as words or as a voice; it was a knowing, an ancient lore that had been passed down through the generations of trees and something known by the Celtic people. It was this insight that shaped Celtic Reiki into what it is today and eventually led me to completely rewrite all the practices I teach.

And yet, more than this, what the tree whispered to me as the world faded away, had a profound effect on how I perceive the world, people, and all living things. It blew away any notion of right and wrong, good and evil. It showed me how to become a new person and it taught me three things about trees:

> Trees, on the whole, tend to have
> an hysterical sense of humour.

> Trees are wise and loving and some of the
> best teachers we can ever hope to learn from.

> Trees make great furniture!

# Two Maples and a Blackbird

As I stood, staring out into space and sensing the tree giggle at the rather embarrassing outcome of the interview, I tried to fathom what had gone so wrong. It was then the deep resonance of the tree filled me with the answer. At first I was puzzled, not grasping the wisdom the tree imparted to me, however by the time the crew had finished the interstitial, I comprehended the vital importance of the Ash tree's message. In fact, if ever there were a reason to sit and stare through my fingers at that masterpiece of television, it would be to simply watch that transition. The infinite passage from unknowing to understanding, viewed in a thirty second piece of 'throwaway' footage.

What I unravelled in the Nuin vibrations was basically the knowledge of fluidity, of how a message can change as it is offered from one person to other. A story, a belief, a snippet of juicy gossip; each time the information is given it takes on a fragment of the teller. Their perspective becomes intrinsically bound with the information, giving it shape and definition. In the earliest, oral traditions of the Celts and other communities, fables, legends and spiritual teachings where not only ancient wisdom, passed from person to person; they were tributes to each and every person that had touched those words through time.

There I was on a beautiful summers' day, speaking to a comedian about something precious and life-giving. I intended to hold Celtic Reiki up for the world in an arena where it could be ridiculed and laughed at and not only this; I was being filmed doing it! I was creating a long-lasting record of Celtic Reiki philosophies, how Essences were harvested and the method of treatment. I was advocating dogma and rigidity in a practice that is fluid.

Each and every tree is an individual, growing to an inherent set of instructions that offer enough space to be unique. Thus no two trees are the same, even if they are of the same species. When we realise this, we also come to understand that each and every Celtic Reiki Master is unique and also works to the same principle of working within the parameters of Celtic Reiki, yet with enough space to breathe and make the practice their own. By standing up as the originator of the system and saying, "This is how it's done", I was closing that space down and leaving less room to grow for future Celtic Reiki Masters. No tree grows well when it is bound and restricted; the same philosophy applies to Celtic Reiki practice.

It was at this point I started to celebrate the gift of originality and sharing my perspective as a testament of who I am, what is more, by doing so I enabled others to be who they are, without judgment or condescension. It was this inspiration that compelled me to rewrite my Usui Reiki practice into what is now known as vReiki. After so many years of being told how it 'had' to be done (in very conflicting ways), I thought it was time to add my own touch to the fluid tradition of Reiki practice. And as my view of Usui Reiki shifted so did the way I styled my practice of Celtic Reiki.

One of the most apparent results of this is seen in how Celtic Reiki Masters view the concept of Reiki, in comparison to those who learn Usui Reiki. In this chapter, let us create a magical place to sit and tell stories about our ancestors and the ancient wisdom that has been handed down to us. Visualise a small clearing in an ancient forest, surrounded by ancient trees that shelter and nurture us as we sit around a campfire. The fire burns brightly, creating a warm glow in the dim light of evening. The crackling fire sends embers into the air and the hypnotic flames dance and enchant as we fall through time to an ancient Japanese Maple forest...

In this forest lived a tree named Usui, of whom, many have expressed their opinions over the years. Some say that Usui was a maple of the most dazzling lime green, whilst others say his leaves were a vibrant red. Some say he was a tree of mighty proportions, whilst there are those who comment on how delicately formed he was. It is suggested that upon entering the forest, one would automatically find one's way to the Usui Maple because of his magnificence, and some comment that the tree was so innocuous that he was hardly even distinguishable from the rest of the forest.

The perspective that many people agree on is that the Usui Maple did discover an amazing method of growing taller than the other trees in the forest. According to the Usui Maple, a tree should practice a connection to the Earth and the Heavens by means of peaceful reflection. It must then use this connection to heal itself, becoming strong and healthy in mind and body. Finally, the tree that wants to become taller than other trees would also use its connection to the Earth and the Heavens to heal the other trees of the forest, by expressing the connection in song. The Usui Maple called his method, 'The Usui Maple Get Really Tall Through Singing Method".

One day, a nearby Cherry tree said to the Usui Maple, "Usui, your connection to the Earth and the Heavens is a wonderful thing. You are much stronger, and all of us here in this area of the forest are healthier than ever. Though, do you think the name of your practice is fitting?"

"What do you mean?" Asked the Usui Maple, rather puzzled.

"Well," replied the Cherry tree, "Your practice has such a magical effect on all of us and I was just wondering if there was a new name that might better reflect this magical effect?"

Usui Maple pondered over what the young Cherry tree had asked him and decided that he would indeed search for a name that instilled the very nature of his discovery. Usui sang loud and long, asking the wise elders of the forest to tell him of the ancient tree lore; mysterious arts that were long forgotten by the younger generation of trees.

Eventually, his song was heard by the wise elders that lay deep within the forest and they sang back to the Usui Maple; their deep, resonant voices narrating the traditional tales of a mighty force which connected the Earth and the Heavens. This force was known as the 'Magical Source of Infinite, Universal Power'!

"Hmm," thought the Usui Maple, "I like that name!"

And so, Usui sang far and wide about the 'Usui Magical Source of Infinite, Universal Power Method' and all the trees that heard his song grew taller and stronger. Throughout the forest, trees began to learn Usui's method and then passed it to other trees. The message travelled even further, to regions of the forest far from where the Usui Maple grew.

The song glided through the far-reaches of the forest, until it came to a dark and lonely area, in the shadow of an enormous mountain range. Here, the sun did not shine, so most of the trees were sickly and weak. They did not care for growing taller, as there was no sunlight here for them to reach towards. However, a maple named Hayashi realised that whilst the Usui Method may not be of use to his community for growing taller, they may benefit from the strengthening and healing properties contained within the song. So, Hayashi Maple learnt how to connect to the Earth and the Heavens and adapted the Usui Method to focus on the healing qualities of the Magical Source of Infinite, Universal Power.

It was the spring, when Hayashi awoke from his winter slumber to find a blackbird perched on one of his branches. The blackbird had a broken wing and cried to Hayashi Maple, "Please Hayashi Maple, use your song to fix my wing, for I cannot fly and I soon will die!"

Hayashi Maple considered this for a while and decided that all life, be it tree or animal was the most precious thing on Earth and therefore, must be saved if there were the slightest chance of success. So, he sung the most beautiful song he could muster and all at once the blackbird was lifted into a beautiful trance. She flew up towards the sun and flapped her healed wing, high in the sky.

"Oh thank you!" She cried. "Thank you Hayashi Maple for healing my wing! My name is the Blackbird Takata and I would like you to teach me your wonderful, life-giving song!"

"Teach you!" exclaimed Hayashi Maple. "But you are not a tree! Only trees can sing the song of Universal Power!"

However, Hayashi Maple had not realised how determined the Blackbird Takata was. For she flew around his branches all spring and summer, singing "Birdsong is as able as the song of the tree! Teach me! Teach me! Teach me!" Imagine that, morning, noon and night!

As autumn draw near and Hayashi Maple prepared for his long winter slumber, the blackbird's constant pestering became tiresome and so he taught her Usui Maple's song. And as winter came and Hayashi went to sleep, the Blackbird Takata flew across the oceans, singing her heart out and telling the world about the joy of Usui Maple's healing method.

Our story does not end here, though, for one day, the Blackbird Takata came upon a group of beavers, who were not interested in trees, except when using them to build dams. As Takata started to speak of Usui Maple's song, she noticed their displeasure and so she changed her story. She told the beavers how Usui was a beaver, who discovered an infinite power that could help other animals to become healthier and stronger and build better dams. She also said that rather than singing a song, the creature must bang its tail to connect the Earth and the Heavens.

The beavers did as the Blackbird had told them and they felt wonderful. They banged their tails against the ground with ecstasy, growing stronger and healthier with every blow of their tail. Some even used their newfound power to build bigger, taller dams, whilst others taught the Usui Maple Method to the deer and fish.

Long after the Blackbird Takata had died, her song of the Universal Power and the two Maple trees lived on in the howl of the wolf and the call of the whale. It can be heard in the squawk of the eagle and the cry of the lemur, the roar of the bear and slapping tail of the beaver. Usui Maple's message of strength, healing and achieving a sense of personal excellence lives on.

The biggest challenge to face the remaining custodians of the Universal Power was yet to come, for after the Blackbird Takata had left the physical world, the wolf began to argue with the bear. "My howl is the correct way to connect to the Power, so your roar is wrong and you should howl like me!"

The eagle said to the lemurs, "My squawk is directly descended from the Usui Maple's song, whereas your cry is not, so you are all frauds!"

The beavers added to the debate, "Remember that we told you all about the Universal Power in the first place, plus we personally knew the Blackbird Takata, so we must be right!"

The whales just listened and when they did, they heard the song of the trees; not only the song of Usui Maple and Hayashi Maple, but also of the elders, who related the traditions and ancient knowledge of the Universal Power. And the whales knew that all creatures have their own song, their own way of connecting to the power of the Infinite Universe. The whales understood that there is no right way or wrong way, there is just your way and my way, of which neither is better or worse. They just are. As the whales watched the wolves, bears, eagles, lemurs and beavers squabble and bicker they wondered how any of them could hear the song of the ancient trees over the noise!

Hence, the whales just continued to call their perspective of the song, in the hope that others may hear it and discover their own song too. So, if ever you want to hear the song of the ancient trees and learn for yourself the Power of the Universe, you only need listen to your own truth and you will find your way.

In this story, we find many parallels with the historical background of Reiki, for example the Usui Maple discovered a connection that he related through similarity to an ancient belief. Mikao Usui, the originator of Usui Reiki (commonly abbreviated to just 'Reiki'), experienced an overwhelming Satori, or enlightenment during a 21-day meditation on Mount Kurama in Kyoto, Japan. By creating various techniques to help others experience their own Satori, Usui originated what he called 'Usui Teate'. Later he revised the name to 'Usui Reiki Ryoho', meaning 'Usui's Reiki Method'. The concept of Reiki was derived from the Shinto perspective of Reiki as a facet of Universal Force (Ki).

Dr Hayashi, who was also pivotal in the transmission of Usui Reiki to the West, had a greater focus on the healing aspects of Usui Reiki, as opposed to Usui's view of Reiki as a path to Satori. Just as the Hayashi Maple was not interested in growing taller, he just wanted to help his tree community heal and become stronger.

The Blackbird Takata, based upon Mrs Hawayo Takata, who brought Usui Reiki to the West, was the first woman to learn the principles of Usui Reiki after pestering Hayashi to teach her. Mrs Takata did indeed alter the historical context of Usui and his methodology to present a more 'palatable' view of Reiki practices.

Whilst Usui Reiki remains a powerful and profound healing method all over the world, it does tend to go hand in hand with the 'in-bickering' and 'my way is the right way' attitude of a few Usui Reiki Masters. Whilst these Masters are in a minority, their effect on the Usui Reiki community often creates a culture where Practitioners and Masters feel the need to justify their beliefs, as opposed to being empowered to nurture their own path and methodology.

Originally, Celtic Reiki was in-part based upon the practice of Usui Reiki, however the events that took place with the Ash Tree, led me to re-imagine the Reiki basis of Celtic Reiki. I did this by going back to the Shinto foundations of the Reiki paradigm and building the philosophies of Celtic Reiki from there.

# I Got The Ki, I Got The Secret!

It is phenomenal how life can change in a moment; a single incident, the blink of an eye, a breath and everything is different. With each step on the journey that creates our lives, we are permanently altered and can never go backwards. We do not unlearn; we can only ever change what we know in the present, when the memory of the past is distorted by discovery of the future.

I have had several such moments in my life; two stand out more than any others. The very first time I looked into the eyes of hatred, and I do not mean dislike or aversion, I refer to absolute, all-encompassing hatred. It is not a memory I conquered easily and the realisation that I was hated by another person produced lasting change in me, to say the least! The absolute antithesis of this was the very first moment of my very first Reiki treatment. For in that infinitesimal fragment of time, I discovered, while someone can regard you with hatred, love, is in every point of every fibre of everything. The Universe is saturated with love and kindness and benevolence, if only you look with eyes of love.

In so many ways, I am grateful for each and every person that has hated me, because they are a reminder to me of how it feels when somebody looks at you in that way. It is because of those feelings that I, myself have never looked at another person with hatred. I've been angry and said hurtful things, I'm not perfect, but I had the good-fortune to discover how easy it can be to look at other people with an all-encompassing love—and as such, to be totally immersed in love.

Reiki taught me about karma and balance. It displayed in that first connection how we do not have to buy into what we know from the past. I've seen so many people who have experienced the hate and prejudice of others, offer hatred in return, when given the opportunity. Perhaps they believe it is their 'right' or that 'revenge' is a good thing; maybe it is the bullied child that bullies an even weaker child. My personal view is that when you're connected to hate, you are connected to it, whether it be through the eyes of another or in reciprocation. Reiki whispered to me a message that is now carved into my very being—it's about what you offer that is important!

It is this understanding of Reiki, as a force, connecting us to an all-pervading wisdom and unconditional benevolence that underpins Celtic Reiki. For me Celtic Reiki is that same loving force, viewed from the perspective of the natural world. The 'Celtic' and the 'Reiki' are merely traditions that help us grasp the overwhelming joy that exists in every part of the Universe. This joy, this indescribable force is so beyond our understanding that we can only hope to catch glimpses of its wonder. The traditions of the Celts and the Eastern principles simply offer tools through which we can discover our individual way of reaching the love for ourselves.

From my perspective, Reiki is one of several facets of Ki, derived from the ancient Japanese concept of a 'Universal Life Force' that creates and supports all life and physical matter. In recent years, the term 'Reiki' has acquired different associations, which often connect it exclusively with the healing practice of 'Usui Reiki Ryoho'. If we turn to the Shinto and Tao philosophies of Reiki we see it could be viewed as the electricity that powers our modern world. Reiki is the force, not the practice as such. In the same way we would not use the term 'electricity' when referring to a 'CD Player', an important distinction exists between the force of 'Reiki' and the practice of 'Usui Reiki' or 'Celtic Reiki', and so on.

Consequently, when we discuss Reiki (and Ki in general), we are examining the force, not techniques that employ Reiki as a source of power. With this in mind we can explore the various facets of Ki, which in modalities of Reiki practice, such as vReiki and Celtic Reiki, consist of Shinki, Ishiki, Reiki, Tsuki, Jiki, Denki, Kuki, Mizuke, Shioke, and Kekki.

Let us begin our exploration of Ki with Shinki (the Divine Ki) which represents pure thought and wisdom that has no physical presence at all. Shinki exists outside of our realm of understanding and no variety of physical material can actually interact directly with Shinki even though all physicality is originally derived from it.

In the traditions of Shinto and Tao, the concept of Shinki is of a force, so omnipotent that it possesses the knowledge of all things, except one. This one, simple hole in the wisdom of Shinki is so imperative that Shinki constructs the entire, physical Universe in search of the answer. With all this potential for experience, Shinki then sets about rediscovering all there is to know about itself, albeit from the perspective of illusion; the illusion of space and time and of being something other than Shinki!

Shinki is perfection, and enlightenment and wisdom; it understands everything there is to know from every perspective and viewpoint. It knows of mountains and love, it knows every star and all the animals. If a place existed or there were a taste or a smell, a colour or a sound, Shinki knows about it. Shinki is aware of absolutely everything there is to know, except what it is not to be Shinki.

Shinki does not know how it feels to climb a mountain for the first time, to fall deeply in love with another and to rely on trust alone that they are loved in return. It has never gazed into a night sky and wondered at all the unknown possibility the Universe had to offer. Shinki cannot feel the wonder of swimming with a dolphin or holding a puppy dog in its arms. It has never tasted chocolate or smelled a rose, never gazed at the vibrant, green leaves of a tree or heard the sound of early morning birdsong. Shinki knows all there is to know, except what it is 'not to know'.

Hence, Shinki made the decision to learn what it was not to be Shinki and devised a complex plan to create the illusion of separateness. Shinki would change itself over and over again, until it eventually forgot its true nature and could thus, find its way back to being Shinki once again. In this elaborate adaptation, Shinki would forget everything it knows and have to rediscover every single experience as if for the first time. As Shinki made the decision to create this transformation, something amazing happened; the very existence of a thought that was beyond the understanding of Shinki, turned Shinki into Ishiki; consciousness.

Each and every distinct perspective, from which Shinki can possibly study itself, establishes a life-purpose. The instant this life-purpose becomes distinct from Shinki, it becomes conscious, and this state of consciousness is the first layer of transformation, from Shinki into Ishiki; the Ki of Consciousness. If we said that Shinki was an idea, Ishiki would be the conscious exercise of creating a blueprint or 'master plan' for that idea.

Ishiki is the act of conscious creation, taking a root life-purpose and constructing an elaborate plan around that purpose. This initial blueprint is multilayered, so that the illusion of separateness from Shinki is apparent. Once the plan is formed it achieves a state of stasis or balance that exists as potential, but not as physical reality. For the next stage in the process to take place, Shinki must adapt once again.

Shinki transforms itself into Kekki (the *Ki of Blood*), which has no intelligence but exists as pure physicality. It is the substance from which the building blocks of life are created. However, Kekki does not have structure and just as its conscious Ishiki counterpart, it exists in stasis until it is combined with a second facet of transformed Shinki—Shioke (the *Ki of Salt*).

While we are striving and moving towards our goals, Shioke is with us, enabling our reflection of the Divine. Shioke is credited with the life span of our cells and our physical bodies, for we only need live as long as we choose to accomplish our dreams; once we have done what we are here to do, we no longer need to exist and so Shioke enables our departure from life as well as our appearance into it.

Shioke is a receptacle in which Kekki resides and while both combine to fashion the basic elements of life, they always retain their respective separate qualities and individual characteristics. Thus, we can regard Kekki as the concept of concrete and Shioke as the idea of a 'block shape'. Put the two together and you have the ability to create concrete blocks. Now that Ishiki has the building blocks of the solid Universe, it sets about assembling in accordance with the master blueprint.

The next phase requires Mizuke (the *Ki of Water*), which is the catalyst for communication and enables the combination of Kekki and Shioke to form complex structures. Mizuke is expansion, reproduction and growth in this trinity of Ki facets. It continually strives to further itself and produce a greater scale of life and physical being. The tenacity of Mizuke is echoed in life, forms the basis of our emotions, sexuality and body awareness.

Mizuke symbolises the energy of a waterfall or even the ocean. Wherever there is water, be it the unyielding flow of a cascading river or the calm of a mirrored lake, we can sense the Ki connected to the movement and essence of water. Our body is composed mostly of water and as such, we resonate with Mizuke at an integral level.

Traditionally viewed as the facet of Ki that binds Shioke and Kekki into greater masses of solidity, Mizuke is responsible for the need to reproduce, to create in a physical sense. It is closely connected to our emotions, which are also formed of liquid, and our physical body: an embodiment of fluidity, flow and the cycle of life.

It is part of the 'human condition' that we are never satisfied with what we have, whether we desire more money, more material possessions, more time, greater wisdom, more from a relationship or even things such as more peace and quiet, we are constantly searching for more...and it is Mizuke that drives us in this search. Just as a stream flows into a river, into the sea, the Ki of Water leads us on a path of acquisition, which can become addiction.

Wherever there is expansion, there must also be restraint, for if these three aspects of Ki could endlessly grow, there would be merely a huge mass of physical matter without boundary or division. So in limitation we discover the diversity of Kuki (the *Ki of Air)*. Kuki is the initiator of boundaries that regulate the growth of Kekki, Shioke and Mizuke. It is these borders that facilitate the concepts of individuality and separateness, as they mask our connection to each other and with all things. Kuki is the facet of Ki that offers the illusion of you, me, them, this table, that chair and so on. In separation however, Kuki also binds us by instilling within each of us a mutual rhythm, a common goal. It is this which drives and motivates us, making us individuals, yet causing us to seek connection with others through our relationships, families, cultural groups, communities and so on.

The synthesis that is created between Mizuke and Kuki is one of balance as we see from the harmony that is created between expansion and limitation, of union and separateness. Just as Kuki proffers the illusion of being detached and alone, Mizuke gives us connection and a merging of all our facets and those beyond our perception. When we understand the way we are connected as a holistic being, that same ideology can be applied to all things, material and etheric.

In the Ishiki plan of conscious creation, there is now the foundation of a solid Universe, expansion and growth, as well as limitation and definition. Ishiki has the infinite scope of all solid matter, with unique and individual qualities to 'act out' the life-purpose of Shinki. However in order for these isolated, separate chunks of matter to interact, there needs to be some form of attraction and repulsion, therefore the creation of dynamics comes into play, with the transformation of Shinki into Denki, (the *Ki of Thunder*).

There are some interesting paradoxes between Denki and Kuki, which start with the idea that Kuki, despite being the Ki of Air, is actually more tangible than Denki, the Ki of Thunder. The second remarkable irony is that the Ki of Thunder is more like electricity and the Ki of Air is comparable to waves of sound.

We could view Kuki as being a noise that is carried on the breeze, or the echo that reverberates along a valley. It is the facet of Ki that is carried on the air. It is the space between all things or rather that which appears to be space. For Kuki is actually an illusion because it is not space, it is force like all the other facets of Ki, yet its role in the bigger scheme of things is to proffer the idea that we are not connected.

Whenever we feel isolated or alone, whenever we limit ourselves or hold ourselves back, whenever we perceive the things we desire as being unobtainable or too far away: it is Kuki at work. The wonderful thing about Kuki is that in division we find unity, in singularity we discover ourselves and in limitation we grow abundance. For Kuki is not only a paradox when compared to Denki—it is a paradox in itself.

Kuki provides us with a mutual rhythm; like a drum beat that we all walk to. In the illusion it casts for us, we are able to develop our own uniqueness or personal power and to connect with the things around us. Philosophers and soothsayers have said that we all want the same things for ourselves, for our families, for our communities. The personal goals may differ slightly according to culture and social factors, but essentially we all want to live our lives, to be safe and be happy. This utopian view becomes distorted when you start to add the complexities of life upon it, yet this is the drum that Kuki beats for us. It is the ability to personally overcome the separateness of life and feel connected that we all strive for. To realise that whatever we strive for, whatever we want is actually within everybody and everybody is actually part of a whole.

As we find connection with each other and escape our isolation, we discover love, the embodiment of Denki. Denki is at the root of all human experience. It nurtures acceptance, although it also has associations with cleansing as it teaches us through fear of loss and heartache. The Ki of Thunder is like the storm that cuts through stagnation and stillness, provoking movement and a purging of the things we no longer require. It is through the lessons of Denki and the love it offers that we strive for our life-purpose and discover the origins of our being here. By following our path and discovering both love and loss on our way, we learn how to experience empathy and compassion: qualities that create Denki.

Denki is a powerful force that is somewhat misleading inasmuch as it is the lightning that Denki symbolises, as opposed to thunder. The term Denki translates directly to our concept of electricity and is thus a potent form of Ki that acts exactly as the electrical force we are accustomed to.

We often refer to the energy generated between two people as "electric" and it is this electricity that really sums up Denki: the force that binds us, drives us and sometimes causes us to fall. Denki is the love between a mother and her child, the sexual energy between two lovers, the bond between life-long friends and the compassion of a healer for the sick. Yet, although the purpose of Denki is to help us overcome the isolation we feel while encased in our illusion of separateness, we very often find that it can make us feel even lonelier. We learn very quickly in life to crave the force of Denki, its physicality makes it seem finite and limited and linear.

This means that, like the energy of money or time, the Ki of Thunder appears to be restricted in the amount we can perceive at any given moment. Thus we have occasions when we feel that we will burst with love, and at others we feel that there is not enough love in the world. It should be mentioned that Denki is not 'love' itself, but the force that is present whenever love, passion or compassion are felt.

Due to its physicality, Denki is very tangible and does offer us rudimentary wisdom. Denki is the twinkle in the eye, an intimate touch of the hand, a beautiful summers day, the laughter of friends, the smile of a baby or the excitement of a dog greeting his owner. It is the elusive, yet special moments that are scattered throughout our days, which affirm we are alive and connected to all things. The innate simplicity of Denki is equalled only by its complexity; the beauty derived from our connection to Denki is matched only by the despair when it cannot be reached. Denki unites us and causes wars.

When motivated by Denki, we strive for the things we need and to provide for those we love. Denki is the great motivator that gives us the strength and ability to attain our goals and walk our life path. Yet, having experienced the joy of Denki in our lives, it creates a huge sense of loss when it leaves us. However, through loss, we learn how to reconnect to Denki by empathising with those who are experiencing what we ourselves have been through in the past. Thus we grow to understand the nature of love in a wider sense, travelling beyond the limits of love for those around us, to compassion for all living things.

Hence Denki embodies the journey of cleansing, washing away stagnation and stillness to form an ever-changing dance of vibrancy, potency and electricity. Denki can be finite or infinite depending on how you work with it. We can learn how to experience what appears to be a limited love, or radiate a never-ending compassion; we can create conditions or offer unconditional love: the choice is ours to make.

As each individual becomes aware of their uniqueness and meaning, they meet others and form loving connections; they develop social groups, cultural communities, large populations and so forth. With people experiencing their own private motivations and priorities, we observe the formation of complex dynamics that need to be supported, directed and, to a certain extent, governed. It is in this function that Jiki the *Ki of Magnetism)* is created and guides us both individually and at the level of group consciousness.

Whenever groups work together to produce or uncover something good, it is Jiki that channels their effort and brings it to fruition. Jiki oversees our awareness on the larger scale, in relation to our society, faith, race and species; leading us onwards, we are drawn together by its magnetism in order to find our unique cultural routes to truth and beauty. It is Jiki that offers awareness to the other facets of Ki discussed so far, thus presenting them with the ability to act together for the unified good of all things. This particular layer of Ki creates a magnetic attraction amongst the other layers, bringing them closer and managing the overall progression.

The Japanese word 'Jiki' can be directly translated to the Western concept of magnetic force and the concept of 'magnetic Ki' is derived from the Taoist view of Life Force. In many respects comparable to the scientific view of an electromagnetic spectrum, the Taoist belief is that all Ki is divided into facets, some of which are adaptable, yet when stable they have a specific and definite purpose.

Jiki is the aspect of Ki that guides us at a group level as well as individually. As people, we are all very different and while we may have much in common with others, we are still unique and individual. With all this contrast and diversity, it would be very easy for us to walk in very different, opposing directions. As each person walks his or her path, they play a part in a huge expansion. An example could be seen as everybody starting in London and gradually walking forwards in different directions—as this happens the group expands in all directions. When somebody reaches Birmingham, somebody on the opposite side of the group arrives at Calais, and so on.

With all the multiplicity of things in life, from science, to art, to spirituality, to health, to love, to business, to personal tastes, we can connect to an almost endless number of personal choices. Each choice is like a village or town on the map we are travelling. With this much to choose from, it would not be long before we disperse so far from each other that we would just dissipate. It is here where Jiki comes into being, for Jiki creates magnetism in groups; a magnetism that binds us together so that we remain close enough to preserve stability as a species and remain in connection with the life-purposes of Shinki.

All groups create Jiki when they begin to disperse as this particular facet of Ki will bring them closer together, while maintaining individuality within the group. This means that we are not only connected to each other through Jiki, but we are also connected to all living things, all places, all events, all planets, all stars, all galaxies, and so on.

As with all magnetism, there is a flipside to Jiki for, in addition to its attractive properties, it also repels. This means that in group-dynamics the same force that keeps us together can also push us apart. As Jiki pulls us closer and separates us, we move forward, driven by relationships, interactions, situations and circumstances. In some instances we may be propelled in one direction at an amazing pace, whilst at other times we may meander slowly on a multitude of paths. There are also occasions when we become 'stuck' between two equal and opposing forces. Here we become still, yet because of the huge power of this divergent force, we are buffeted and impacted from both directions.

This means that as we interact and move in relation to the overall dynamics of our family, social, community, geographic and biological groups, we will also be influenced by our location within these groups. Those at the centre of the Jiki sphere of authority will move in line with the group, whilst those at the fringes will move in their chosen direction, either leading the group, or opposing the group. Those leading will often be held back while the group 'catches up' and at anytime the group may decide to move in a different direction.

Of course, there are times when an individual disagrees with the group or discovers an 'unconventional' way of doing things. When this occurs, two possible outcomes are available: the individual separates from the group and moves to another 'sphere of existence', or the group likes this 'new' way of doing things and moves with the individual in this new direction. This entire process is done without communication at a conscious level and happens under the natural dynamics of Jiki.

If we examine these dynamics more closely we see that Jiki is, at any moment, directing a very complex dance of attraction and repulsion. It is moving things towards us and pushing other things away. For the most part these interactions are 'internal workings' and can be seen superfluous to the overall dynamic. However, when we work with Jiki, we can not only influence it to a certain extent, but we can also read its dynamics and flow.

The effect we have of consciously entraining the attractions and repulsions is often known as 'manifestation' as we can draw what we want in life towards us and remove the situations/circumstance that we do not want. The reading of Jiki dynamics is known commonly as 'psychic ability'—we not only say what has happened and what is occurring at this moment, but also what is about to take place in the future.

Jiki usually exists on the very boarders of consciousness. We are aware of its actions and consequences, but direct interaction with Jiki is usually reserved for those who are said to have special gifts or natural abilities.

Awareness of our Jiki layers of perception connect us to 'Tsuki', (the *Ki of the Moon*). If we imagine that Ishiki is the consciousness of Shinki (Divine purpose), then Tsuki is the consciousness of the physical world. Tsuki reflects the Ishiki design in the same way as a skyscraper reflects the architect's blueprint and creates the closest parallel to the concept of a soul.

Tsuki is the pinnacle of physicality and spiritual achievement before we cross a bridge into the non-physical realms of Ishiki. If we imagine the darkness of night, when daylight is gone and we can easily lose our path, Tsuki can be perceived as the reflected light of the sun that helps us find our way. If ever you have been out walking on a moonlit night, you will understand just how bright the moon can be. Tsuki represents our spiritual expansion and the recreation of life-purpose in the Physical world. Tsuki is a sense of inner-mission, which is sometimes referred to as 'fate', though it can be affected by choice.

There is a fine balance between human experience of 'the other side of the bridge' and the reality of the other side, which means that the boundaries can become nebulous and we may even get confused between our experience and the bridge itself. Of course, the bridge is that of Reiki, or (the *Ki of Spirit)*; a connection between the pure wisdom of Shinki and the material nature of the other facets of Ki.

I used to speak of Tsuki and Reiki as the same entity, however I felt there needed to be a distinction between Reiki as a force and our human experience of Reiki. For, interaction changes things—just as we are irreversibly altered by our conscious experience of Reiki, so Reiki is altered by its experience of us. Tsuki is that transformation from the 'Universal' to the 'Experiential'.

Traditionally, Reiki is the organiser and equalising force of life that accomplishes its aim by balancing all facets of 'physically orientated' Ki. In creating equilibrium, Reiki heals and offers enlightenment. With a highly *intelligent* nature, Reiki understands the physical being in a way that Shinki cannot and hence acts, through Ishiki, as representative of the Divine in our physical world.

Many believe, when in balance, the facets of Ki create perfection of all things, yet if these different layers of Ki fall out of alignment, we soon see the development of disease. This filters down through each aspect of Ki, from Tsuki through to Kekki. A lack of spiritual fulfilment leads to mental and emotional unrest; social and cultural issues arise from this discordance, we feel cut off, abandoned and alone. When this happens, we try to readdress the imbalance by focussing on physical solutions, relying on addiction and co-dependence to compensate; this in turn leads to physical disease.

Reiki rebalances all the aspects of Ki by bridging the gap between physical and spiritual, using the knowledge of Shinki to bring the physical aspects of Ki back into alignment. By re-establishing balance, Reiki heals us on all levels and creates a path for us to find our personal connection with the Divine Ki: our own relationship with The Source.

# Come Away, O Human Child!

*"…To the waters and the wild,
With a faery, hand in hand,
For the world's more full of weeping,
Than you can understand."*

W.B. Yeats

The dominion of fairies and of elves is veiled in mystery and ancient tradition. For whilst most people in modern, Western society confine the creatures of the 'old lore' to realms of fantasy, there was a time when these ethereal beings were much feared and revered. Their names were never mentioned just in case you attracted their attention—something you really did not want to do!

If you were unfortunate enough to catch the eye of 'fey-folk' you may get away with the inconvenience of having objects moved around your house. However, should you arouse the interest of some castes of fairy, you may have your children stolen, changelings running around your home and in really extreme cases you may well experience a slight case of death!

To our ancestors (and particularly our Celtic ancestors), the fairies were immensely powerful creatures that might destroy lives on a whim; their only motivation being, because they could. Now, some fairies were benevolent and therefore helped people in various ways. Some were completely indifferent to humankind, ignoring us when possible and only interacting when forced to. Many, however, were the absolute epitome of 'yuckiness' and actively sought out the joy of playing pranks, stealing and generally being nasty, whenever the opportunity was presented to them. These quintessentially yucky beings were so awful that is was felt better to avoid fairies all-together than risk the unwanted attentions of a wife-stealing, child-swapper!

On occasion, I have met people who would gladly throw open their windows and call out fairy names at the top of their voices, if they thought this might have their partner taken away, or their children swapped, (though in pre-Roman days, people generally had the idea that valuing your family was a good thing).

So with the notion of: family—good and 'yuck-fest'—bad; how did the Celts express their connection to the beings of spiritual layers? We certainly know they worshipped very different deities to those widely accepted today, we also know that the Celtic tribes had their own beliefs about the elves and fairy-folk that frequented their land, forests and homes. Who and what these various idols were, however is very much a mystery. With the breakdown of oral tradition and the evolution of very different lifestyles, much information about Celtic spirituality has been lost.

Apart from a very few carvings and images, the Celts never wrote or described their spiritual beliefs in static form. This, as I learnt the hard way, was to prevent the creation of stagnation and dogma. The power of fluid and adaptive oral-history provides a way of adapting the most valuable lessons to the needs of ever-changing communities, however when traditions are overwhelmed by written language, they can also be easily lost.

This is a theme that permeates the modern perspective of Celtic theology, inasmuch as an oral tradition enables an interweaving of contrasting and even conflicting views. The very nature of verbal communication means that information can be adapted, nuanced and tailored to the needs of every listener. The written word simply produces an incongruous body of work, which openly displays its inner-conflicts in a rigid and unchangeable format.

This is not intended as a criticism of the written word. The ability to communicate through textual means has offered humankind immeasurable growth in education, historical awareness and technological advancement to name a few. The issue is that writing things down is like a rock to the conversational river. One is fluid and ever changing, the other changes slowly and over long periods of time.

With spirituality and energy, change is even faster than the flow of water downstream. Even verbal transmission is cumbersome where energy is concerned—just think about the time it takes for thunder to be heard after the lightning has stuck—and now imagine how useful the newspaper headline "lightning is striking now" would be! That is the challenge of writing down any aspect of energy work or spiritual art—by the time it is written and committed to paper, things have changed!

In terms of an intellectual pursuit, written debate is an excellent way of exploring Celtic spirituality from an academic point of view, however, as far as the actual beliefs and philosophies of the Celts, I believe that practise based in energy is the closest we can get, followed, at a distance, by oral traditions based upon those practices.

Hence, when it came to intermingling Celtic philosophy with Reiki practice and the Essences of trees, I focussed more on the wisdom of trees, the guidance of higher knowledge and commonly available information, as opposed to relying too heavily on clandestine texts or secret tomes.

Interestingly enough, this valuable lesson of trusting what I learnt from the trees, subsequently made it possible to apply identical lessons in relation to Reiki philosophy. That is, I turned away from the mammoth body of Usui-orientated and highly speculative texts and focussed more on an energetic interpretation of beliefs.

I feel it was working with these principles that have led people to call Celtic Reiki a rediscovery of Neart (also known as Nerth). The concept of Neart is actually comparable to that of Ki, Chi and the other forms of 'Universal Energy/Force' and is viewed as the Celtic 'version' of this infinite force.

Whether Celtic Reiki is the reclamation of a lost power or simply the reimagining of traditions for a modern world, I would not like to speculate. What I do know is, Celtic Reiki has offered me parallels to the stories of legend and folklore. And, through my own experience of the world from a Celtic Reiki perspective, I have sensed things on my own terms that mirror the realms of fairy and elf.

One of the most tangible experiences is a connection to the horned one. Initially, I wondered if this figure I kept seeing in dreams and meditations was Herne the Hunter and certainly that was the name that kept popping into my head. Later I started to recognize these images as Cernunnos; Celtic God of the Woodland.

There are various associations between Herne and Cernunnos; however they are believed to derive from very different sources. Herne has strong connections to the Buckinghamshire area of Britain and Cernunnos is centred on what is now the Paris region of France. Also, the mythology surrounding these two iconic figures is very different, however the blending of symbolism and perspective around the horned figure often leads to the conclusion of them both originating from a single entity or source.

The stag-horned figure has long held associations with darker times for me, personally. My earliest memories from about the age of two or three, are haunted with the dark, terrifying images of dangerous entities attempting to come through the window of my bedroom. For a child to be afraid of monsters is not unusual. Indeed, the majority of adults I have spoken to, will tell with delight, their childhood dread and recollections of night-time denizens coming to get them!

I find it quite amusing that the most horrifying imagery from my infancy now holds such joy and wonder for me. Flashbacks of a dark, ominous shape looming above my window, its gnarled branches silhouetted against an orange, sodium lit sky. The frenzied group of horned creatures that scraped across the glass, as they jostled to get in. And the most horrendous, the bat-like demon that towered into the sky, watching me with malignant, yellow eyes. Each of these creatures would send me screaming into my mother on a nightly basis, however, the image of a gnarled tree, stag-horned beings and dark, yellow-eyed entities now possess strong bonds to benevolence and immense personal power.

You see, I doubt that the images I witnessed as a child were of the solid world; whether they existed anywhere outside of my imagination is up for debate. Although, I do, personally, believe these entities exist on some level of consciousness and I also have faith in their desire to nurture and guard me.

Why do I believe this? Well, Celtic Reiki has guided me down a rather unusual path and along the way, I have met some interesting characters. Some of which seem the stuff of legend, some the imaginings of a children's storyteller and a few are just downright nonsensical. However, all (whether they are actually otherworldly or merely unconscious metaphor) have offered me life experiences beyond anything I could ever have imagined and make talking to trees seem extremely 'conventional'.

Fairies, elves and other nature dwellers need no rhyme or reason for acting as they do. Capricious in loyalty (if they even know of such a thing) they often act in any given situation based on the disposition of their caste. So, a Dryad will usually show benevolence, unless they have experienced some heinous cruelty in the past, or they sense danger. Brownies are for the most part, loyal and affectionate creatures, particularly if you show them kindness. Pillywiggins are giggly and flit from flower to tree to person, as a butterfly does. The Elven castes are notorious for having a problematic relationship with us humans. And, what are traditionally known as 'demons' (and I call 'Reflectors') can be terrifying! I shall cover the Reflectors further, when we speak about my years as a Psychic Medium.

One thing that I can state without a doubt, from my perspective is that if you are compassionate towards the trees and the natural world in general, the fey will recognise this and reward you for it. Now, in fairy terms, 'reward' may mean not causing a slight case of death, but it's a start!

For me, a typical journey through the forest will reveal many otherworld dwellers, from the Dryads (tree spirits) to Watchers (tall, thin creatures that never interact, but 'watch' from a distance—hence the name). Pillywiggins (think Tinkerbell) are usually aplenty, as are Deva (the sentient energy beings of plants and creatures). You may come across Fragments (spirits or ghosts that represent some unconscious facet of yourself), various forms of Guardian (those who nurture and protect an area or individual), or Shape-Shifter (a diverse range of entities that alter their form to blend in, test, or deceive).

If you become aware of the forest dwellers, it is because they actively want you to recognize their presence or to interact in some way. Watchers or the non-interactive forms of fey-folk are usually sending out a message 'not to trespass', to 'be vigilant', or simply to let you know that 'you're being watched'. Although, when Celtic Reiki Masters happen upon watchers, they are usually just acknowledging the Master's presence, rather akin to a 'professional courtesy'.

When the entity you encounter wants to interact, you will often understand very quickly, the reasons for the meeting. It could be a 'you're not welcome', or possibly a 'I want to know who you are and what you want!' In which case, you will feel foreboding, fear, or some form of sharp stabbing pain. When I encounter this type of entity, I simply walk away. Do be aware that if you are a Celtic Reiki Master already, forest entities may treat you with kindness, even if your arrival is not welcome. When you encounter these situations, be aware of the nuances in the vibrational communication and take your leave. If you ignore the polite requests to move on, you may end up with the harsher response!

Conversely, the creature will often just be curious about you. They will want to know more, maybe to learn, or to find out what your reaction is. Frequently they wish to initiate some transaction or exchange. I'm usually overwhelmed by the amount of interactions I have on a short woodland walk, particularly in an area I've not visited before. It still brings a tear to my eye, when I am reminded how excited the trees and the fairy realms are about Celtic Reiki.

I feel so genuinely privileged on occasion, when beings from the otherworld, present me with an extremely rare glimpse into their realm. I was on a quiet walk through a Cornish woodland one day, when a couple overtook me on the path. Just as they were heading out of sight on a bend ahead, a Watcher walked right passed me; his 'legs' as tall as my whole body. He acknowledged me and my awareness of him and sped after the people in front. For me, this was as real and as awe-inspiring as the first time I interacted with an Orca or every loving gaze I've ever had.

Each time I meet a new Dryad or Pillywiggin, I have a tendency to do that "aww" thing, young children do. The sight of a grown man acting in this way in public is quite a spectacle in itself! Yet, in order to interact with trees and the fey-folk, I am very happy to make a spectacle of myself. I've harvested tree Essences under the watchful eye of ancient beings and woodland deities, I have alleviated the pain of the sick and wounded with the assistance of magical beings, and I have been able to show my fellow students how to experience these and many other wonderful experiences for themselves.

Some may think that it's all in my head, but you know what? I really don't mind. I have experienced such joy and overwhelming happiness through my connection to the natural world and the otherworld that any criticism fades into nothingness. Besides, anybody who believes the Universe only exists on layers that can be quantified by our five senses or technology based upon those five senses is like the person who lives in a cave and says nothing exists outside.

Think of the smell of a fragrant rose and the blue of the sky, the sounds of a babbling brook and the taste of a creamy hot chocolate and then imagine a dark, dank cave. That is how I perceive the comparison of experience between living in a sceptical, limited world and discovering the art of Celtic Reiki. However, you just can't explain to a nine-year-old how complex and important loving relationships are—they have to discover that in their own time.

When reminiscing about all my adventures through the otherworld and linking these to the Celtic philosophies I have collected along the way, I realise that I have been stolen away by the fairies, not in an actual, physical sense or in an 'away with the fairies' manner; I am completely enchanted by the privilege and wonder, the knowledge of their existence has given me. This feeling of belonging is far more valuable and integral than a lot of what the physical world has yet to imbue amongst individuals and society in general. Though I have never felt the need to wander away permanently with a fairy hand in hand, the enchantment for me is holding open the door so that others can peek inside too.

# The Little Christmas Tree

One of the most poignant times for me, in the creation of Celtic Reiki arrived in a very small bundle of plastic netting and took the form of a three foot tall Christmas Tree (Norwegian Spruce). Celtic Reiki has always held the core message of caring for our tree friends, with the knowledge that they act as custodians of our planet. Little did I know what was about to transpire and how forever my basic outlook on life would be changed over the next few months.

Imagine a world with no trees or other plants. A wonderful aspect of the human mind is that you can envisage situations and scenes that cannot be. For, whilst you are capable of imagining a world without trees and plant-life, you certainly would not be alive in that world. The plants that inhabited our world before animal life came into being, spent millennia preparing the world for us. Their daily routine of converting the toxic atmosphere into the most basic element of animal life (breathable air), was carried out over a period of time far beyond that of our existence on the planet.

I'm sure the trees did not do this 'for us', however, in the bigger scheme of things, the trees actions were necessary for our creation and eventual inhabitation of the Earth. Since humans came into being, though, we have used trees for fire, shelter, tools, etc. and whilst this was initially done with great respect for the tree-kind, in modernity we have come to view trees as commodities, which only live to serve human needs. In fact, the majority of humans do not spend that much time thinking about trees at all.

To a certain extent, trees have a very different view of life. They accept the cycle of creation and destruction, life and death. From what I can gather, their belief is that when the physical tree dies, the tree lives on through the offspring and the other trees in the forest. Yet, if you ever experience the pain of a tree that has been chopped down, it does not feel that way.

As friends stood on the doorstep, beaming with joy at the gift they had bought me, I did my utmost to hide the horror I felt upon seeing the Christmas tree they brought. A few days earlier I had made the mistake of commenting that I wanted to buy a tree to decorate that year. In my mind this had been an artificial tree or a potted tree that could later be planted and offered the opportunity to grow. Out of sheer kindness, my friends had purchased the tree from a vendor outside the local supermarket and thought it would make a wonderful decoration.

When they had left I quickly unwrapped the tree from the netting, placed him in a bucket of water and sat with him for several hours. The sensations that pervaded the very air around me, were of absolute, gut-wrenching fear. Severed from his roots, the tree knew he was dying, but this young, innocent creature was so new to the world that he had no concept of what was happening.

The overriding image the Christmas tree instilled in my mind was one of a child, around the age of four or five, battling to understand a terminal illness and doing so, without the support of parents, guardians, or even friends. He was completely alone and terrified.

Those first few hours, I spoke to him in the Ailim tongue. I listened and learned and I took time to simply sit with him 'in' his fear and guide him to a place of feeling calm. During these long hours, I could discern no difference between this little life that ebbed away and the life of any other creature. I truly empathised with the notion of life as a precious, fragile force that is beyond price or measure in the material world and is so bittersweet in its performance.

I allowed my mind to meander through possible ways of saving the little Christmas Tree, from attempting to take a cutting, to the rooting of his severed trunk. I could see no way of saving this life and even in the weeks to come, as I researched to various methods a transplanting trees or fusing trees together, I was at a total loss. Therefore, I simply did what I could energetically for my new friend, from offering Reiki treatments and dosing with various homeopathic remedies, to just sitting and talking to him or listening to him tell me about his hopes and dreams.

As time passed, I learnt much from the Christmas Tree who changed from a terrified, infant tree into a very profound and spiritual being. As he recoiled from the shock of being cut down by humans, only to find acts of kindness offered by another human, he was presented with a conundrum. It was this challenge that taught the Christmas Tree how to love those who had treated him so horrifically—and taught me the nature of forgiveness.

Christmas Tree faded over the period of several months. I watched as his needles gradually turned copper-brown and fell out, his tiny trunk and branches became dry and brittle, but I knew he was still there.

Everyday there were intangible differences to his vibrations; he was more expansive, less fearful. These changes were more discernible as weeks passed. The slight processes of daily transformation were more pronounced over longer periods. He was wringing every drop of experience from his little corner of the world, propped up in a black bucket of homeopathic water, watching the world walk onwards. And as he absorbed all he could, he grew wiser and less focussed on the physical world.

I would sit with him often, with no need for words or purposeful interaction. Just sitting and sharing the experience of proximity; of being close to each other. As his body slowly failed him, I thought that he would grow weak, yet his energy perspective became stronger as he became detached from the solid world.

It was this growing vigour in Christmas Tree's spirit that taught me not to fear death. No matter how the body weakens and fades, the spirit and energy of living things can never die. If anything, the processes that form the death of a physical body, intensify the spirit. As spring turned into summer, I witnesses the most profound example of how energy cannot be created or destroyed—it only changes from one form to another.

It was a day in July when I stepped out into my garden and sat beside the little copper-coloured frame of Christmas Tree's body that I knew it was time to say goodbye. The sun was fierce that day and I knew that with the summer only halfway through, he could not drink enough through his severed trunk to survive very long in the heat. I asked if he would like to come inside the house for a while, an attempt to keep him here a little while longer. As I felt him slipping, I so desperately wanted to keep him with me, yet when he replied softly, it was his time, I knew he was right.

I sat with him for the longest while as he whispered the precious secrets of his fleeting life, his observations and his discoveries. He requested that I use his body and the vibrations that emanated from it to create a remedy, like those I had used to help him through those months of coming to terms with his fate. I agreed and inside of me something broke.

It seems somehow ridiculous to feel so bereft over a little collection of twigs and dried needles, yet this is the next lesson I learned from my friend. Nothing, absolutely nothing, no matter how seemingly small or insignificant deserves to be thought of as worthless. All life, even the most minuscule organism is important and can teach us valuable lessons. Even the inanimate object that is regarded as sentimental or imbued with personality can be a source of immense connection and love. From the gift, given with joy to the teddy bear that is held tightly in the arms of a child (or an adult). It is the connection and the feelings inside that matter. Love is love, whether it is for a gift, a toy, or a pile of twigs.

I spent a little time with the Christmas Tree, offering him a Reiki treatment and sharing some last, poignant stories about the great Spruces and Pine trees that I had met. The lone Fir tree and the many conifers that had helped me create the Ailim Essence of Celtic Reiki. I had, of course, told him these stories before, at a time when he listened with the excitement of a young child. Now, he just listened and I knew his spirit was longing for a different place; a faraway place.

Eventually, I had the impression that he wanted to be left alone and so I whispered goodbye, one last time, stroked his upper branches and left him to enjoy one last afternoon in the sunshine.

I quietly watched over Christmas Tree from a distance, at several points throughout the day and each time he gave the impression of an old man, staring out to sea on his last day on Earth. I believe that if he had eyes, they would have been focussed on some far off shore, passed the horizon. The next day when I ventured out into the garden, he was gone.

It was several months later, I bought myself to a place where I could work with the twigs and leaves that were left of my closest tree friend. I lovingly created a mother tincture for the Ailim Celtica homeopathic remedy and sent this off to the Helios Pharmacy to be 'potentised'. I carried around a small piece of branch so that I could feel him with me. I would cry a little, each time I saw the empty bucket, standing in the corner where Christmas Tree had been.

When the homeopathic remedy arrived back from the pharmacy, I hurried opened the packaging and held the tiny bottle of Ailim Celtica 6c—and once again, I was reunited with the little tree as he was in life, like an echo that returns to source or a memory that becomes clear once again.

Here was another lesson Christmas Tree had for me to learn; knowing that death is merely a transformation into some other form; understanding that energy (and the perspectives we create of it through consciousness) is eternal and infinite; I realised that we are retainers of knowledge—we keep the memories of those we love alive and we pass on their insights, so others may learn and discover joy through the wisdom imparted. I learnt that a man can be the source of life for a tree and that a tree can remember a man long after he has left this world.

I understood totally that every tree I offered kindness to, sat and spoke with, protected, or nurtured would remember me and the knowledge I communicated. This information would then be spread across forests and generations of trees, so if somebody else, somewhere in time or in some other place was ready to listen, the trees would tell them the lessons I could teach. And I knew that I was not the first to realise this!

Many people, throughout time, from different places and of different cultures, also recognised the tradition of trees to whisper among themselves about those of benevolence and kinship. Thus, if I wanted to learn about Celtic wisdom or the ancient mysticism of Reiki and other facets of Ki; if I wanted to speak to ancient shamans and soothsayers and creatures beyond human perception, I need look no further than our arboreal cousins. They all had many secrets to tell…if only I was willing to listen.

# The Nameless Tree

Elated and excited about my new understanding of the teachings from Christmas tree, I found myself faced with a new challenge. Having discovered valuable, new beliefs about death (or rather the transcendence of death) I was now faced with the concept of terminal disease and an entity that systematically saps and eventually kills any tree it touches.

The Unhewn Dolmen Arch or nameless tree, has long divided opinion, because of its parasitic nature. Known in modern times as Mistletoe, the plant is believed to be one of the most sacrosanct and revered trees of the Celts. It was held in such a sacred light that it could not even be named—for naming the tree would be to limit its extensive and infinitive power. Unhewn Dolmen Arch roughly translates to 'the blank Ogham' as it is represented in the Celtic alphabet as a single line, with no staves. As this was certainly cumbersome, the tree was informally known as 'all-heal'; so renowned was the Mistletoe for its abilities to cure all disease in humans.

Birds, such as the Mistle Thrush, eat the sticky, white berries of Mistletoe and then deposit the seeds on the branches of a host tree. The seed sends suckers and eventually roots into the branch of the host and it develops into an adult plant by using the nutrients supplied by the tree. Mistletoe that is unchecked and spreads will eventually weaken and kill the host and it was this predatory nature of the Mistletoe that caused me (and many others) to regard it with mistrust.

Over the years I have spoken to many people about the Nameless Tree and many express opinions very similar to that which I once held. Even some of the druids I have worked with in the past had reservations about the parasitic nature of Mistletoe. Druids possess a very deep spiritual connection to the plant and use a golden sickle to harvest the most blessed of mistletoes: those growing on the branches of an Oak tree.

It was not until I was led to work with Mistletoe, both in dried and homoeopathic form that I found myself completely amazed by the power and spiritual wisdom of this very peculiar species of plant. Sensing the energetic potency of the Unhewn Dolmen Arch enabled me to understand why the Celtic people revered it so much. So I set about working with the Mistletoe and the various species of host tree in order to discover what the trees feel about this curious creature. I was astonished by what the trees told me.

Trees provide us with an amazing elucidation of the way our Universe behaves. Naturally, this is simply a single perspective, yet it has helped me to come to terms with some of the most incomprehensible pain and suffering I have witnessed. Anything that can help us to grasp the greater design or bigger picture, brings us nearer to a resolution. Just as the understanding of how a disease works can help us find a cure, whether that be from a scientific perspective or the holistic approach. Curing the disease is the priority, not the validity of the ethos used. The trees teach us that with a slightly different perspective of the world, we can transcend all kinds of hardships and hurts.

The attitude of many trees towards Mistletoe, not only gives us an alternative perspective to the intrinsic core of disease, it guides us to the very essence of life and our experience of it. For whilst trees, on the whole, fear the infestation of All Heal, many recognize the necessity and the wider perspective of a value beyond the physical sacrifice they undertake.

Therefore, in spite of the parasitic affect of Mistletoe in a physical arena, the spiritual implications of the Unhewn Dolman Arch are infinite; as it has the power to create enlightenment for the host tree. By choosing to accept the Mistletoe, the host is offered in return, such wisdom and 'energetic ascension' that it becomes a far greater being. The host gives a little of itself away to evolve far beyond that of any single tree.

On a purely physical echelon, trees (the quintessential emblem of our natural world) spring from the Earth with strength and singular focus. They rise upwards to the heavens and then splay outwards in search of the life-giving energy of sunlight. Yet they never lose their deep connection with the ground and the remembrance of what it is to be 'of the Earth'. As an organism, trees are like any other corporeal being; programmed to produce offspring and to survive, individually and as a species.

However, once those physical needs are met, a tree may often realise other priorities, including the experience of life on layers that are beyond the physical. This spiritual nature of trees cannot be explained by science or logic. They are one of the most fundamental forms of physical creature, though the complexity of their introspection and reflection from their own perspective is immense.

This is a quality that humankind shares with trees, albeit, from a very different perspective.

Assuming that a tree develops in the ground and survives external influences, such as disease or human intervention, it usually lives for a long time and only ever sees the world from a single place. These are some of the factors that create a spiritual yearning in the spirit of trees.

Conversely, humans migrate, witness great change, and rather than adapting to their environment, they fashion and adapt their surroundings to meet their needs. This very different methodology also creates a desire for knowledge and wisdom; the quest for why 'it' is the way 'it' is. This spiritual imperative within us does not derive from the physical being—it is a synthesis that is beyond the Earth. I tend to look at it as the place where the sunlight hits the leaves of the tree; a dance between two very different layers of reality.

The Mistletoe represents a plant that is parasitic in the physical perspective and yet, symbiotic on 'cerebral' and spiritual layers. It provides the host with opportunities to experience what it is, not to be integrally connected to the ground. The Mistletoe never touches the ground, unless it grows so large as to reach the soil, or it falls for some reason. The aerial nature of the All Heal is revered in Druidic philosophy and provides benefits that are far beyond the host's understanding. However, the host has faith that the spiritual insight it gains and the greater, Universal viewpoint are worth the sacrifice.

Just as little Christmas Tree discovered the beauty of a world without roots and grounding; as he discovered the joy of being cast adrift into a world of fear and pain and death, only to be brought to the person who would love him, deeply; all trees which give a home to the nomadic Mistletoe discover similar wisdom.

It is this spiritual evolution that is held so sacred among those who possess a resonance with the natural world and our tree friends alike. In narrow physical terms the whole situation points to a horrible end, however, when we account for the spiritual perspectives involved with the Mistletoe, we see the same unexplainable compassion that leads a spiritual leader to express love for his torturers, or the innocent man to forgive his accusers for their naivety.

For me, the realisation of these insights initiated a vast journey, seeking connection to Mistletoe and the trees that host this enigmatic plant. My adventures led me to deep respect for the host trees and a sense of awe for the Unhewn Dolman Arch that is unlike any other form of plant that I've encountered.

Initially predatory in feel, the vibrations of Mistletoe are more akin to a carnivorous animal as opposed to plant-life, however, very different to meat-eating plants like the fly-traps. As one diverges from the physical layers, the sensations of the Mistletoe Essence appear to pull away from the ground; heady and disorientating. Then, there is a sense of something alien; and I use this word in as a conveyance of the utterly indescribable vibrations that appear to be 'not of this Earth'. Everything that grows on the planet is connected by a shared perspective, yet the Mistletoe is deficient in this and it creates the feeling that the Mistletoe has blundered into our reality by mistake or as if it is somehow 'misplaced'; a schism.

After many months of connecting to and harvesting the female-gendered Mistletoe, I came across a male of the species in a car park. And I was astounded by just how different the two genders are.

The male was greater in peculiarity than the female plant and, as I have learnt time and time again with Celtic Reiki practice, the more diverse an Essence is, the stranger (and more profound) the lessons that accompany it are! This particular form of Essence sent me on a journey into the realm of dis-ease and the power of the human spirit.

The years I have worked as an Energy Therapist and Teacher have presented me with the privilege of meeting amazing and courageous individuals; those who have experienced unimaginable disease and trauma. I have spent time with people who are facing various forms of cancer or some other disease. On occasions these have been disfiguring or completely disabling, and in some circumstances the disease has been fatal. I've met those who are conquering life-threatening addiction or the most hideous of life experiences. I have witnessed the sheer strength and determination of those whose world has fallen apart. Most of these remarkable people all know that time is the most precious of all commodities, and no matter what we have or yearn for; time is a rare and finite energy.

I personally believe that energy is infinite and eternal—we live in an abundant Universe, where anything is possible. The challenge for everyone is—the definition of energy is finite—and herein lies the issue. The existence of the physical body is created from definition, the experience of life through that body is definition, and each person's life experiences are definition. All of which are so immeasurable, yet so unbelievably small. Every smell, taste, sight, sound, and sensation creates a further definition in our lives; every idea or thought; every leaf that grows or blood cell formed; each a new parameter within an infinite

Universe that longs to be defined; just as Shinki yearns for knowledge of itself, our Universe is formed from definitions created from within its own unlimited potential.

For all these parameters and description, one seems to be the most finite and limited for all living things: time. The most precious commodity we have in life and in so many ways, all we have to offer. For how we spend our time, creates our own unique definition of the Universe.

Christmas Tree taught me the value of each and every single second. When we realise that death is imminent, we slam on the brakes as the inevitable approaches; knowing that we just cannot stop in time and all we have is a few moments more. I've seen that same message resound in the eyes of the dying and the lost alike. And through listening to the reveries of each person along the way, I've glimpsed how important all memories are; how we need to treasure every fleeting fragment of joy and pain from the moments we have, even if we have a lifetime's worth still to come. For there is never enough; not when the foot touches that pedal and we brace for impact.

Despite the vast diversity in the people I have met on my journey, many have expressed identical needs and have comparable perspectives on their situations. Dignity and respect are often essential; very few people want to be treated like a 'thing' or an object to be prodded and poked and subjected to invasive treatments. In addition to these essential aspects of conduct, there is often the need for an acknowledgment from those unaffected by disease or trauma that they simply cannot understand what 'it is like'.

As somebody with an integral need to help others, I wanted to find a way of ensuring my empathy was not misplaced. Many teachers and practitioners feel they know best and therefore close themselves off from new experiences or adaptation of their knowledge. I did not want to 'know best'; I just needed to move closer to an appreciation of the most important factors for the people that I encountered.

Subsequent to my exploration of the Unhewn Dolman Arch Essence, I started to focus on how each person expressed their situation; as opposed to what I assumed they 'must' be feeling. My attention clicked into noticing the relationship many people articulated regarding the disease, trauma or situation they were confronting. I knew that I was ultimately destined to glean my own perspective of other people's circumstances and emotions (as opposed to their actual feelings and situations). However, I realised this may help me be the best I can be, as a therapist and teacher and most of all, a person.

Some of the discussions I have had over the past few years have mirrored that of trees with a Mistletoe union. One person spoke of his drug addiction as if it was a companion that walked through life by his side. The addiction was not feared or reviled, even though it had decimated his body. The drugs and addiction had taught him about his own determination and inspired him to vanquish physical, emotional and psychological challenges that most of us could not even imagine or grasp to any meaningful extent.

He was an unquestionable hero; a champion of human spirit and experience. The 'drug addict', who some may deem the dregs; an outcast or undeserving of kindness, I believe, had made choices that took him to a place most of us would never go. His voyage to that place had also given him an unwavering belief in himself and his capacity to overcome the darkest of times. Every day he made conscious decisions, which many never have to make and could not cope with if confronted with them, without similar experiences to evolve their perspective. There are people who may question why support is given to people like this man; I imagine those people have not died twice and clawed their return to a world that had shown them so much hatred and bigotry.

I grew up, surrounded by this kind of intolerance and prejudice at the time when HIV/AIDS first came to the mass attention of the Western world. Having known and worked with a number of people who are HIV+ I have witnessed in total wonderment, the sheer force of people who keep living to the full, in the face of hatred and stigma. That's before we even come to consider the retrovirus! Yet it was here that I have heard people talk in the closest analogy to Mistletoe.

Many people I've known with HIV/AIDS talk about their 'knowing' of their infection, before being tested. As if some intuitive connection to the virus is made before the conscious confirmation is apparent. Thus, they embark on adventures through experience, be these of life events, psychological battles, spiritual awakening or a finding peace and acceptance of who they are.

The upshot of these expcriences is often a realisation that life is not about hatred, prejudice, the views of other people, or their bigotry. It is about choice —the choice to make every single moment memorable and enjoyable; to live (and sometimes die) with dignity and to seize every single second in this physical world with a love that transcends life—be it a love for oneself, for those close to us, or for people on a wider scale. It is the very existence of that love that counts, not where it is directed.

The Unhewn Dolman Arch teaches us that when we face our greatest challenges, we are never more alive. If we slip into the domain of disease or encounter hatred, we become ambassadors that pave the way for others, so that their journey may be smoother. By doing so, we create wisdom that transcends the physical world and takes us on to an alien place; the future and the discovery of the unknown.

For me, the Mistletoe Essence is not about a parasitic relationship or the sapping of life—it shows us, when we are so integrally grounded in the Earth, we occasionally need to give a piece of ourselves to the air (or spirit) so that we can learn to see beyond the solid world. The Unhewn Dolman Arch gives dignity and respect to all of us, for we all know pain, the pang of isolation and what it is to be misunderstood.

Through my adventures, since harvesting and evolving the All Heal Essence, I have attained a great respect for my own body, the fragility of time, and the immense value of health. I have witnessed miracles and developed a deep sense of compassion for all people, regardless of who they are or the choices they have made. I am now very aware of how assumption or lack of care can hurt, and how what most people believe is an acceptable way of treating each other, is actually incredibly degrading to others, but mostly to themselves.

Believe me, there have been many times when I ached to the absolute core of my being, and pleaded not to be the one learning these lessons. However, when I am introspective about my accomplishments, I realise it was because I experienced those dark times that have benefitted people across the globe. I then begin to ask myself, what would the world be like if each and every person could see what I see? What if we all knew the value of unconditional love and had the determination to implement that prize in our lives, each and every day?

An Oak tree views the forest through the perspective of Mistletoe and cherishes each moment and each creature and each encounter with an unwavering and total commitment to the experience. If we could all learn how to emulate this, without the need for pain and suffering, imagine the difference it would create. Take a moment to think about your life and if your pain was everybody's pain; if we all stood together to transcend that pain, how would you feel? Well, I consider the suffering of each and every creature to be the suffering of the Earth—and we are all of the Earth.

# The Psychic Years

Even though I retired from Psychic Mediumship in 2008 I feel Celtic Reiki practices have influenced my psychic abilities to such an extent (and vice versa) that our journey in the grove would be incomplete without some reference to the psychic experiences that contributed to Celtic Reiki development.

The field of psychic work is very closely related to energy work and in particular 'energy medicine'. The intuitive sense that one learns through working with a therapy, such as Celtic Reiki is very close to the experiences attributed to the professional Medium. These two realms are so similar, in fact, that when pioneering a professional level psychic development course, I actually based the whole syllabus on the healing arts! My belief being that we all have psychic ability, locked away deep within us and hidden by lack of confidence, fear and a barrage of other limiting emotional-associations.

I had learnt through my years of originating energy arts that we have the abilities we need, albeit hidden and very often atrophied through neglect or lack of use. The secret is to heal the emotional barriers and remove the blockages that stop a person from realising they actually do have the abilities and voila! They light up with talent in whatever they want to achieve.

In retrospect, I am now quite sceptical towards the area of 'paranormal phenomena' inasmuch as that what we regard as psychic ability is actually a perfectly normal, human ability that most people forget to use. The idea of there being anything scary or clandestine about what psychics do is very often a method of control—whether this is conscious or unconscious. This debate is better left to another time, however, when we understand that the psychic ability simply means; the awakening of innate cerebral and spiritual abilities, it becomes a lot more approachable.

There are several main junctures in my life where Celtic Reiki and the psychic realms have intersected; from the creation of several Celtic Reiki Essences, to how my tree friends supported me in the rather stressful role of a Public Event Medium.

It was my instinctive, intuitive ability that guided me to work with the Lone Tree and thus originate the first Essence of Ailim. My 'psychic skills' were with me every step of the Celtic Reiki journey, whilst defining Essences and constructing a methodology of testing, practise and teaching the newly found modality. Yet, it was not until my experiences with Sanctuary Oak and the refinement of the Duir Essence that the psychic layers of perception become distinct in our Celtic Reiki story.

The initial Duir Essence was created when I assisted three young Oak trees in Mid Wales. These trees grew in a small outcrop of rocks between a river and a quiet, lonely road. All three were very sick and the obvious signs of disease could be seen in the colour of their leaves and the condition of their bark. I treated the trees in turn, over several days and the Essence was formed as a natural side-effect of these treatments.

When I came upon Sanctuary Oak, however, the idea of expanding the Duir Essence seemed immediately to be a virtual impossibility! This large, imposing tree regarded me with what I can only describe as disgust as I approached; I was later to describe his demeanour as 'austere', though I believe 'hostile' is more fitting when describing his attitude.

I stepped up to his trunk and simply asked if I could help in any way. He did not reply at first and then the words, "This place is sick, heal it!" came into my mind.

Upon asking for clarification, the same command was repeated, so I decided to take a look around. The Sanctuary Oak grew at the entrance to an ancient grove near Bodmin Moor in Cornwall. The grove was split in two by a single-track road and was bordered at either end by small groups of houses. Over time, I came to know the grove very well and spent many hours with my tree friends there. My first few weeks working in the grove though, were very dark from an energetic point of view, mainly due to what I was about to discover.

I crossed the road and headed into the larger part of the grove, passed several Rowan and Hazel trees, an Elder and a group of Oaks. As I headed further into the grove, I found myself heading into clustered of nettles and on one occasion, I needed to backtrack because the nettles, thistles and bramble were so dense. Eventually I came to a power line, which cut across the far corner of the grove. Cables that carry electricity overhead can be particularly damaging to the natural environment, especially from a vibrational point of view. The research into occurrences of cancer in people living near pylons also seems to support the view that power lines have some major effects on their surroundings.

This, I concluded, must be the source of the 'sickness' and so I decided to return the following day with some homeopathic remedies. These might heal the effects of the electricity cables overhead and restore vibrational harmony, if only temporarily.

I turned back, in the direction of the road, and made my way along to makeshift path, which was created from two deep tractor-tyre prints. About halfway along this path, something distracted me; a compulsion, or strange, magnetic force pulled me to the right of the tracks. Within seconds, I was back into high nettles and wild branches of brambles that reached head-height.

I don't know why I felt the need to press on through the onslaught of stabbing, stinging things, but I just knew I had to head to a particular spot. Gradually, I came to a clearing and was able to peer through the undergrowth to an additional, but smaller clearing, fifty or so feet in front of me.

To my surprise a woman was standing in the clearing, facing me. She was bolt upright, but her eyes looked down, or so it seemed, as her matted hair fell across her face. Her clothes were very 70's in style and seemed tattered slightly, muddied and just struck me as 'wrong'.

I watched for a while, knowing that she was not actually there in the solid world. She held an arm across her stomach and shivered with cold. I took a sharp breath in, as one does when one recognises what is about to happen, but hasn't consciously processed it.

Her head snapped upwards and she looked at me through strands of black hair. Her eyes burned into me for a moment, and then she spoke.

"I was raped and murdered by two men—and this is where I was buried!" She pointed sharply to the ground beneath her feet and then vanished. And with that my head was flooded with images of these two men, a white van, plastic sheeting, names, addresses, dates and then blackness. I glanced hastily around, to see the ground turning dark, as if a cloud was passing overhead, but there were no clouds on that day.

The lumps of granite, which poked through the mulch and woodland plants, grew dark also. The trees seemed to shrink into themselves. Something was coming; some force or creature that was threatening and malignant to its very core. Off to my left, a dark shape moved through the trees, getting closer and taking the light away as it came. This entity, this malevolent, ominous thing was not of the corporeal; its ancient presence regarded me and I knew it was sizing me up. It gazed into my heart and my mind, searching for weaknesses in preparation to strike.

I've encountered demons (Reflectors) a few times in my life and there is one trait they share: when they attack, it comes quickly and sharply. There is very little time to react and any active assertion on the part of the target must be achieved through prior rehearsal and practise, so it is achieved instinctively. Hesitating for a second, to decide on the best course of defence gives the assailant all the time it needs to be upon its victim. And here is the chilling thought—the reason for this is because, at the very moment you become aware of its presence, it means the Reflector has already begun its attack. The only course of action at that point is to assert the conscious mind, so that you keep control of the situation. Without this conscious assertion, it is easy to panic and then the entity can create havoc.

Intuitively, I reacted to the offensive, using the trusted techniques I have acquired over the years and as I did, I felt it bounce away for a moment, before surrounding me once again. I remained calm and centred myself with steady, deep breathing. The Reflector seemed to ripple through the air about me as it changed and transformed its tactics. You see the aim of using the term 'Reflector' for the entities, traditionally referred to as 'demons' is because I believe the feelings, reactions and sensations they inspire do not come from some outer evil—they come from within the 'victim'. Reflectors feed on your darkest emotions and as they feast, they also reflect those emotions back at you. Therefore all you can sense when in the presence of a Reflector is your own most horrifying fears and torment.

This overwhelming onslaught of emotion is so effective at stunning the focus of the Reflector attack, because it is so integral to the focus personally. Anybody who has vertigo will know how the panic grabs hold when on the highest floors of a tall building, or how deep-seated the fear of spiders can be when one is crawling up your leg. These are the varieties of fear and forceful emotion the Reflector uses to paralyse its prey.

The only way I can describe a Reflector connection is like a crack that sounds in the air around you, as if the very oxygen is igniting with electricity. It is fast and all-encompassing and it until you get use to them, they are terrifying. Of course, the most important thing when you stumble upon a Reflector is to remain utterly calm and composed, no matter how close it seems or how much you want to run. Your breath becomes slow and regular and from deep within, for it is this serenity and focus on the core of your being that asserts your vibrational field.

It is often taught in psychic training that a shield, cloak, or bubble is the best method of 'protection', however I favour visualisations that emanate from the very centre of one's being, projected outwards to form a sphere of assertion all around the body. I have come to prefer this method, since I have heard so many people with basic training talk of how the entity 'takes the cloak (etc.) away'. The entity cannot take away something that is part of you, which stems from who you are and is integrally you at a basic level.

Another tip that I recommend to all my students is to use the word 'assertion', instead of 'protection' wherever contextually possible. My rationale for this clever use of linguistics is down to the association we have with the two words. Unconsciously you protect yourself against things that are usually bigger than you and very often are unknown or unquantifiable in some way. You assert yourself against equals, such as other people. As soon as you think of the processes of protecting yourself, you place yourself in the weaker position and your unconscious mind reacts accordingly. When you assert yourself, your unconscious believes that you are facing an equal; suddenly you feel much stronger and your energy work explodes with effectiveness.

As I asserted my inner calm around me, the formidable attack of the Reflector began to fail and slowly recede, back into the grove. As it ebbed away, the light returned and I walked to the road as quickly as I could.

The very next day, I started to research the names and other information attained about the young woman's murder, however I could not find any verification of the incident. So I began to explore my options in relation to previous day's experience. The woman, the murder, the granite, the reaction of the trees, how the Reflector had made its appearance, the electricity cables and so on.

Gradually a picture began to emerge of a place ravaged by mining in the Victorian era. Electricity pylons and high levels of radon from the granite causing a field of vibrations that lowered the frequency of energy about the whole location. A history of violent crime even? Well, to this day I have not been able to track down any mention of the woman I saw that day, however I have subsequently had intuitive messages about sacrifice and a long history of violent attacks on the land that is now the grove. Perhaps the repetitive cycle of violence, combined with the vibrational 'miasma' created the ideal hunting ground for the Reflector who now stalked this place. I planned to return later that day and face the Reflector again, although this time, I would return at night, because I knew that under the cover of darkness it would reveal itself completely and I could get a better idea of its strength and power.

Cornwall has a rugged and sometimes bleak landscape, which is atmospheric at the best of times. On occasions when the mists roll in and the twilight falls upon the land in a particular way, there is an incredibly mystical feel to the place. This is something shared by all the Celtic locations; a tangible sense of lands that are home to ancient, enigmatic beings and lore, which transcends our everyday world of solidity. The Cornish landscape is tinged with history and tales of smuggling, ghosts, and all manner of strange beasties! When you're preparing to spend a night facing your most visceral fears in the shape of a demon, the secretive ambience of the Cornish countryside is never more apparent.

I padded my pockets with various remedies, worked on some energy cultivation techniques and prepared to venture into the grove. The setting sun heralded a strangely beautiful sky; so many wonderful shades of colour, yet such a deep sense of menace. As I travelled to towards the moor, I could not shake the distinct impression that 'it' knew I was coming and was looking forward to our encounter with malignant glee.

As I arrived in the grove, the last glow of sunlight was faintly apparent in the western sky. I could immediately feel the Reflector's presence, nearby, yet restrained by an unseen, benevolent force. I decided this must be the trees of the grove, assisting in the only way they could. Remembering the vibrational dampening effects of the electricity cables and rocks, I knew they would not be able to hold it for long. Thus, not knowing how much time I had, I hurriedly prepared.

I did not have to wait long before the darkness came. It was a moonless night, yet the blackness was unnatural, as if the last remaining light was being sucked from the very air. This is quite a common phenomena, associated with locales of paranormal activity, which denotes an entity absorbing the ambient energy to produce physical presence. The Reflector did not give the impression of have definite locality; it appeared to emanate from every rock and even from the ground itself. Like a fog that appears so gradually as to creep up on the unsuspecting traveller, the dark materialised from the very space around me, casting me into a complete shroud of black.

I felt the space around me vibrate with energy, clawing and permeating my senses. It started with fear and I soon found thoughts popping into my head. Worries, memories, motivations came, one after the other. Like the act of flipping through a rolodex, the succession of random concepts flashed through my consciousness, attempted to provoke a response and then faded away when I did not react to it. I knew the Reflector wanted to incite some form of emotional response, so I ignored my internal monologue as it expressed, with escalating determination that the ideas flooding into my head needed attention, as they were extremely important.

You see the reason 'demons' are traditionally renowned for being so effective at what they do is because the vibrational field they emanate, shakes loose all the 'stuff' a person really needs to heal, but pushes it away from their conscious focus. The reason these outstanding 'miasms' remain hidden is down to how they make us feel when we actually acknowledge their existence—as if there is something 'demonic' all around us! It's no mere coincidence that we speak of our 'demons' in relation to what we perceive as 'negative' past events.

One of the things I have learnt when interacting with the Reflector-style entity (or any entity, with the intention of interacting in some way with a person) is their only power is that of suggestion. They cannot physically harm you or 'talk' directly to you. What they can do is immerse you in vibrations that motivate you to make a specific reaction.

People use this principle a lot too. Have you ever been in the company of somebody and just wanted to be away from that person? Maybe, you have found the opposite, where a person draws your attention and stirs a sort of fascination within you, just by being near. These are the unconscious responses to something beyond physical perception. It is the same methodology the Reflector (and other entities) uses to get a reaction.

I once conducted a Psychic Event with a group at the Edinburgh Vaults in Scotland. There we encountered an entity that creates the dynamics of isolation. As a group we were very strong, vibrationally, so the entity's goal was to separate and explore us individually, so that it could find the 'weakest spot'.

Throughout the night, people would wander off, linger behind the rest of the group and even started bickering and squabbling amongst themselves; anything to escape each other's company. I found myself needing to assert repeatedly—"don't wander off" and "stay together". Now, if you were in a location of high paranormal activity, in pitch-darkness at 2am and the Psychic Medium said for you to stick together as a group, would you actively desire the need to separate from the group and go sit by yourself? This is the vibrational strength that entities can muster.

Back in the grove, the Reflector was suddenly all around me; bombarding my senses and thoughts with emotional triggers and vibrations of energy that motivated me to be afraid, to run away, to cry out, to give in. I focussed on my breathing and did not make any action without calm and rational thought first.

I focussed on projecting a series of Essences from deep within myself. Taking my conscious attention to my lower abdomen (The Dantien) and breathing each of the Essences outwards from there. The combination of the inner focus, breathing and combination of Essences was simple enough to think about over the vibrational chaos, yet simple enough to keep my attention.

I selected three Essences that are particularly effective against vibrational disturbances. From the vPsychic toolkit I decided on Salt and from Celtic Reiki, Luis and Tinne. I basically kept cycling these for a minute at a time. I felt the grasp of the being diminish slightly, but then I felt one of the Essences faltering.

Each time I switched to Luis, the Reflector grew stronger again. I slowly and systematically searched for reasons as to why this might be the case, using my breath as a way of keeping calm. I gradually realised that the predominant tree in the grove was Rowan and therefore was a vibration the reflector had great familiarity with. As this became apparent, I knew the Reflector was using a skill that I call OOPS (Out of Phase Shift), which is when an entity or energy worker will basically reflect an Essence back on itself (this can only happen in instances where the person or being using the OOPS technique knows the Essence inside-out!)

I then swapped Luis for a combination of Onn and the vPsychic essence of Silver. This caused the Reflector to lurch away from me, repelled by the bright, vibrant Onn and potent Silver mix. As the sensations of pressure and fear and panic subsided, I continued to focus only on my breathing and the Essence cycle. And, I was glad I did, for moments later the entity swelled up, around me, clawing and shaking at the air all over the place with immense force. Everything became darker than ever, so dark in fact that it was as if nothing existed outside of my head. I held out for a few moments more, holding on to the rhythm of coloured lights that rippled through my vision as all else began to slip away.

Then it was gone, receded away into the ground once again. Snapping back into full consciousness, I started to toss more vibrational remedies to the ground, sealing in the weakened being. This long battle that was more of an internal struggled against my own fears, emotions and thoughts, as opposed to a physical fight, had cost the Reflector much. Its energy depleted, it would now be unable to re-emerge through the vibrational barrier I had scattered across the ground.

I returned to the grove on several occasions over the next few weeks, repeating the laying of remedies and projection of Essences to restore the grove's vibrancy, as much as possible. This dedication and commitment to the place and to the trees that lived there, eventually led to the harvesting of Sanctuary Oak and many other Essences from my friends of the grove.

Harvesting Essences and repatterning areas of woodland are not the only times Celtic Reiki and psychic skills combine. When I worked as an Event Medium, demonstrating psychic abilities to groups of people at locations of paranormal activity, I called upon my Celtic Reiki abilities a lot. You see, when you are an Event Medium, the idea is that you stand up in front of the group and basically tell them about the experiences you are having at that moment. This might be regarding ghosts and spirits at the location, messages or historical information that you pick up vibrationally.

This can put immense pressure upon the Medium, as they are being tested, not only physically and mentally (most events last the entire night, which means working at 4am, usually in icy cold and damp environments!) but also to your confidence. Many of the groups they face are sceptical or want the Medium to prove your ability in some way. Even the most fervent believer in psychic ability may need some 'proof' that you're any good at what you do.

On some events you may have members of the group who have been drinking, are out for a laugh and generally muck around, or who are disruptive in some other way. Whilst these people are usually in a minority, add to their presence a location that does not have much activity or is quiet for some reason and you find yourself standing in front of thirty people with nothing to tell them and a historian/host who is waiting to historically verify the information you express!

This was the situation I found myself in at St Briavel's Castle in Wales. It was bitterly cold and dark, the castle itself was very low on the activity front and we had a particularly large group of people. Internally, I was struggling to connect to any valuable information and had no clue of what I was going to say next. So, as we walked around the grounds, searching for something, anything, I connected to an ancient Oak tree that stood in the grounds and simply asked in the Duir language—"please help me!"

"A person was murdered by my trunk, another hanged from my branches. There are three men standing over there and watch out for the dagger!" The tree replied.

I stood for a moment of recollection, quite dumfounded by the helpful nature of the tree. Then I started to explain to the group what the tree had told me—I should mention, at this point, that while the majority of people attending paranormal events can accept you talk to dead people, the idea of talking to trees denotes that something is seriously wrong, so between you and me, I didn't mention anything about the Oak's assistance.

As I spoke, the tree began to offer details about who the people were; why one man was murdered and the other hanged. I was told where the dagger was buried, names, dates, and so on. The historian, started to verify each piece of information, sometimes historically and on other occasions explaining that other Mediums had also given similar details as I. The one thing that could not be verified was the dagger, though I believe that if somebody were to dig around the area of the tree, they might discover an ancient dagger, hurriedly buried.

# A Lord of Thorns

One of the most majestic and powerful trees that I have ever had the pleasure to meet is the Lord of Thorns. She not only offered us the gift of the Tinne Essence in Celtic Reiki, she also permitted me to create the 'Tinne Celtica' homeopathic remedy, which is one of the most vibrant and joyous remedies I have ever experienced.

I've always viewed the Lord as a mother figure—she is protective and kind and always helps those who ask for her guidance. The wisdom she has imparted to me over the years has been inspirational at times, joyous at others, and on some occasions she helped when nobody else could. The thing I love most about this beautiful tree is the slight sense of bemusement she shows for the strange humans. I imagine her smiling about our funny ways and nonsensical actions, because from her small field on Bodmin Moor, she has a different view on life.

The Lord stands in an area covered by low Bracken and despite her diminutive height of around 12 feet, she towers majestically above all else in the stone walled field. Nearby, gorse, blackthorn, and hawthorn grow, all stunted and gnarled by the fierce winds that blow from the Atlantic Ocean up, to the moors.

Since the harvesting of the Celtic Reiki Essence of Holly it has been a tough time in many ways for the

Lord of Thorns, with harsh winters and dry, hot summers, she has had a severe battering from the elements, yet still she stands strong on the lonely hills of the moor.

Having seen the world through her perspective, she has become one of my most valued teachers. I now realise that it is life itself which is important—not the form that life is packaged in. Yes, the human body is more sophisticated than some and our minds are capable of incredible things, yet the true sign of power, and the greatest, is the ability in choosing not to use it. Hence, the truest lesson of the Lord of Thorns is that of respecting life in all its forms and appearances—of loving our planet and everyday being grateful that the Earth has chosen to support us through another night and granted us another sunrise.

The Lord of Thorns' perspective tends to dominate the Tinne Essence, as I have spent more time with her than any other holly tree. In fact I am reminded of her, each time I pass holly trees in the forest or when walking along the street. The influences of her perspective can be recognised when connected to other Essences too; for example Staif, Ioho, and especially Gort all possess the Lord's wisdom. Harvesting Essences of trees and plants, in the physical vicinity of her magnetic vibrations, saturates the energy with her perspective.

And this is one of those fascinating aspects of the Lord's personality; her ability to imbue things with simplicity, whilst grounding them in the everyday world. You see, I have a longing for knowledge and wisdom, which has spurred me onwards for most of my life. Studying the unusual combination of Quantum Physics and English Linguistics in my twenties, gave me a hunger to know as much as I could about these and similar subjects. Even when training, practising and teaching therapies and personal development methods, I discovered a particular allure surrounding how energy work was perceived in relation to language (and how we think), and when studied through the filter of Quantum philosophy.

These two subjects have played an extensive part in the origination of many techniques, in particular with the incredibly advanced Viridian Method. I was very much in the thick of pioneering VM during my most frequent visits to the Lord of Thorns and she was fascinated by my constant stream of elucidation on the different styles and tools that I was creating.

What makes VM so challenging and so miraculous is the multi-dimensional methodology, required when using it! Concepts of space and time are insignificant and energy work takes on new layers of potential and power. It does, though, take a while to master and is intended for those who are passionate about energy development, as opposed to people with a passing interest.

The Lord of Thorns found VM fascinating and would like to communicate about the philosophies and latest discoveries at length. She would also bring me right back to Earth by reminding me that whilst we can work with energy on emotional, cerebral and spiritual facets of being, we do need to function as people in the physical world.

Therefore, I would regularly be asked to get involved in games with the Lord as she taught me the importance of anchoring inspiration in the solid world. There was one particular thing she enjoyed and that was to beckon me late at night, especially in the harshest of weathers.

Trees and plants recognise that energy exists beyond the physical and can thus, connect to us at a distance, without physical contact, and on different layers of perception. So, should you need to communicate with a tree friend, you do not actually need to go to where they are and place your hands on them, to achieve this. That is, of course, unless your name is the Lord of Thorns.

I have a reputation, amongst some of my students, as a bit of a disaster area when it comes to the natural world and weather—particularly when in combination! Maybe this is due to conducting courses on high hills during sheet lightning storms, or almost plummeting from high mountains on several occasions. Whether it is falling trees, getting trapped in bogs, being rolled up hill in gale-force winds, slipping into icy cold lakes, or a whole litany of similarly bizarre episodes, I've been there and bought the tee-shirt, inappropriate footwear and kagool!

Yet no meteorological-related incident (or otherwise) has been as frequent as my treks across the moors to visit the Lord of Thorns. Whether it be 2 in the morning, with hurricane winds, floods and lightning, or an occasional apocalyptic event, the Lord would call me to give me some profound piece of wisdom.

This was no wild-goose-chase, however, on the occasions when I did venture on to the moor to visit the Lord, I would be greatly rewarded with a gem. The unique approach, adopted by the Lord, however, was unlike other trees, she insisted I go to her, instead of giving me the information remotely or when I had actually been to see her earlier that day! In many ways, she reminded me of a grand old lady, who would summon some minion, so that she may wax lyrical about old times and reminisce on a life almost lived.

## A Lord of Thorns 129

What is more, I came to cherish and respect everything the Lord told me, because I had to work for it. She could have easily bestowed her wisdom upon me, each and every second, if she had so wished. However, giving me the run around (up, down, along and under), instilled a core value in the wisdom she imparted. It engrained her messages deep within me, affecting me on many levels.

The interesting thing is that many Celtic Reiki Masters have suggested similar circumstances with regards to the Lord and the Tinne Essence. Obviously, she does not request a pilgrimage to her location from an American or Australian Master (though give her time!), but there are often tasks to be completed or puzzled to be solved. Exertion of some kind seems to be prerequisite, yet the effort that one puts into the Tinne Essence, one gets back in ways that transcend words and wonderment.

The last time I visited the Lord of Thorns was shortly before I moved from Cornwall. It was, in contrast to so many of our previous meetings, a beautifully sunny day with very little breeze. At the time, I did not know this was the last time I would see her for a while, so there were no long goodbyes, no tears, or words of farewell. And that's the way it should be, for the Lord has lost so many of her friends and whilst parting is a wrench to the heart, I am never far from her in thought.

In retrospect, I think she knew that it would be our last meeting for a long while, as there was a tinge of sadness to her vibrations, yet also a sense of joy. From her place on the moor, she could see a long way and I believe she saw amazing things on the horizon…

# Trouble and Straif

The Blackthorn is the most remarkable species of tree, something I did not fully appreciate until more recently. For me every individual tree holds a unique place in my heart. Every tree I have met on my journey and each new friend I make has their own personality and perspective of the world. Some are wise and knowing, some playful and socially aware. There are trees that remain aloof and austere and trees that seem otherworldly; having an air that can only be described as serene. I've connected to trees that have very little to impart, those who have changed my life with their profound wisdom and those that can gossip a day away.

Yet, the Blackthorn had remained a mystery to me throughout my Celtic Reiki journey, because in all honesty, I was unable to fathom their nature. The Ogham character for the Blackthorn is Straif, which is pronounced 'Strife' and is said to represent exactly that – our conflicts and troubles. Ideally I would assume that the Straif Essence would thus, assist those who are encountering some form of trouble or strife in their current situation. Nevertheless, this just did not feel right to me. I was missing something and my attempts to connect to Blackthorn trees never reached full potential.

It was not until I chose to embark on one of the hardest adventures of my life that I discovered the true potential of the Blackthorn. Before that particular epic is explained, let me assure you of a few things; the first being this; balancing the solid world and the extreme reaches of sensory perception is a fine juggling act that involves a fair amount of experience! To clarify this, let us say that the issue exists not with the solid world, or even the ability to travel to the most exotic areas of energy perception; it is the connection of the two that creates the challenge for most of us.

For a start there is the challenge of describing concepts that are complex and convoluted. Often there are no words to define an experience in energy and when words do exist, they are inadequate to present a full, rich and accurate definition of what is out there (or in there) to be discovered.

The next challenge is the curse of knowledge – which represents the communication of knowledge (from a place of knowledge) to somebody without that knowledge. We cannot 'un-know' what we know, so when attempting to describe our experiences, we assume it is easy to understand. A mathematician may understand Differential Calculus to be simple, so when they explain it to a student who has never heard of the subject (in what the teacher believes to be basic terms), the student has a 'brain meltdown', because they are still trying to finish writing the word 'differential'!

Then there are 'knowledge gaps', which are the 'differential', between what you actually know and what you 'think' you know. We all have knowledge gaps and it is not until we stumble upon something that shines a direct beam of light on to our knowledge gaps that we can see them. For example, when I attended my Usui Reiki One class, I had a magical and amazing day, where I learnt about Japanese Gods, my Shamanic Totem Animal, I picked Angel Cards and drank Aura Soma. It was a beautiful introduction to Usui Reiki and inspired me to take it further. I decided that I knew about Reiki practices, so chose to move forward quickly. I did this by attending an Usui Reiki Two workshop that made we completely reassess what I thought I knew. The same happened when I did my Mastership and when I started teaching – a total re-examination of what I thought I knew, in the realisation that I knew very little!

I soon learnt that we never know all there is to know about a subject; we are on a continuing voyage of exploration and discovery. Nowhere are knowledge gaps more apparent than with vReiki practices, because to understand just how much more advanced vReiki is, you need to have completed an Usui Reiki Mastership class already! Those who attend their vReiki One without any prior experience, believe that is just the way Reiki practices are. However, the practitioners and masters that I have worked with, spend most of the classes saying, "I never knew that!" and "That was never explained before!" and my personal favourite, "I've always wanted to know why that is…now I do!"

The upshot of language shortfalls, combined with 'curses and gaps' in the knowledge department, in addition to a whole range of other factors around definition and complexity, leads us to the conclusion that creating a tangible, practical and usable form of energy art, based on the 'raw' experience is something that takes practise. When I now look back on my early attempts, such as the first iteration of Celtic Reiki, I wonder how I ever knew so little!

As part of my adventures in energy, however, let me share with you something else I have learnt along the way. As I started to explore the most advanced reaches of human potential with the Viridian Method, I came across a collection of universal secrets so powerful and transformative that they can change a person instantaneously and irrevocably. Many of these secrets, I came upon in seemingly random ways, although I know there is nothing random about it! These secrets changed the way I view the world in such an integral way that I have been able to guide myself through life and help others in very tangible ways.

Yet, each time I attempted to explain my most profound discoveries to others, something would stop me – like some mysterious unheard rule that forbade me speaking or writing about these core secrets. I presumed this was down to the aforementioned gaps, curses, and language issues, so knew there was a lesson worth learning on the horizon!

The deep, secrets of the Universe just are...they are neither good nor bad, they have no preference for who you are or the lifestyle you lead, they are just beyond the usual parameters of human perception. However, some people see these secrets as a frightening undermining of their humanity, whilst others are set free by the discovery of one or more of the secrets. Some believe the secrets are works of fiction (fanciful delusions), while others understand them as a profound truth. There are those who would stop at nothing to prevent the secrets from being openly available and there are those who know that, eventually, these will no longer be 'secret' and will change the way humankind exists.

At the time I was unaware that I had also gained the attention of some pretty dogmatic forces that would stop at nothing to maintain the silence about my newfound knowledge. In the background they stirred and schemed to halt the secrets from being introduced into the physical world. People were lined up, ready to play their parts and I, blissfully unaware of what was about to happen, continued to plan and create my most beloved work. It was not until it all fell apart that I unravelled a complex and tangled web of limiting beliefs, most people simply understand as reality. It was then I discovered...these secrets are just the beginning!

The best way to ensure nobody listens to what a person has to say is to discredit them. If their voice is perceived to be that of somebody who was deemed unscrupulous, who in their right mind would listen? Hence, I began to experience a litany of assaults on my character and integrity, in what some have referred to as a 'vendetta'. Organised by a handful of people, most of whom were completely unaware of what they were actually involved in, yet it still affected me badly at the time.

No matter how much time passes by, in what manner we mature with age, or how wise we become, the child within us never disappears completely. They may fade into the past or become lost within a wide miscellany of memories, yet they never truly leave us. Some people spend their lives attempting to move beyond the pain of their childhood years. Some become obsessed with the recapturing of youth, while others frown upon anything 'childish'. For me personally, the preservation of a child-like attitude has given me so much delight, because it means every moment of life may be filled with wonder and joy, if I let it.

Children have a tendency to imbue their surroundings with energy and fantasy and possibility. From teddy bears that come to life, to a cardboard box that becomes a time-machine, or a blanket that is a secret camp. The potential for adventure is never far away and when something magical happens, a child will often embrace it with everything they are made of.

As an adult I have climbed high mountains, talked to trees, battled demons, swum with whales, met beings from other planets and dimensions, and seen the future, to mention just a few quests. Some people may question the 'reality' of these things, but the reality of each of them to me has enabled me to help others change their lives and heal their lives and create considerable happiness. Therefore, the 'reality' of these ventures can be measured in the smiles and giggles that would not be here if it were not for those events.

The blind-hatred I now faced in this situation invited me to cast aside my intentional, child-like view of the world. It encouraged me to give into the threats and walk away from all those years of research and wisdom I had gleaned from a higher source. The fellow that gave me hope when it all fell apart was a tiny Blackthorn tree, who taught me the reason why the Celts named these beautiful little trees, Straif (Strife).

It was a blustery day on Bodmin Moor when I walked up to a twisted, gnarly tree with black bark and long, sharp thorns. I had never noticed him there before, which is unusual for me, but then if trees want to go unseen, they will. The Lord of Thorns had directed me to connect to the little Blackthorn tree, informing me that he would help me to discover the answers I could not find for myself. As I approached and placed my hands amongst his sharp spines, he seemed to move slightly, thus ensuring that he did not harm me in any way, with those awe-inspiring spikes.

Immediately, I was connected to my first day at school, on the first playtime of my life. I sat, alone, not knowing anybody and not really sure what was happening. I watched the other children playing and wished that I could join in their games. I was roused from watching my classmates by a sudden, sharp pain radiating from the back of my head, the shock of which caused me to spin around. I was confronted by one of the boys from my class, who was holding a wooden skittle. He looked at me, without expression or feeling and then walked off. I never knew why he had hit me with the skittle – I doubt he could explain why the incident had happened either. What I do know is this cruel introduction to school life set a pattern that was to continue for many years and become a recurring pattern in my life.

I pondered this for a moment, until the Blackthorn's gentle voice resounded in my head. "You survived!" he said. And he was right; I did survive that first episode and several after. Many of these other events began to flash before my eyes. Disappointment, shock, betrayal, sadness, loneliness, rejection, pain, violence and hatred, tumbled through my awareness like some bizarre and distorted Disney parade from Hell!

There then came a message, very clear and specific, as spoken in my inner voice. He said: "Remember that the sun is always shining – even when there are storm clouds overhead and everything appears dark and foreboding, it does not mean that the sun is not there. Before long, the same winds that ushered the clouds to us will blow them away to reveal the sunlight once more. Even the darkest of days offer some of the sun's rays; for there are no clouds, no matter how dense, that stop every beam of light from breaking through. Every day is filled with light, because we would not be able to see the clouds if the light was not there."

The message was accompanied with an Essence, so profound and potent that it sparked a period in my life that appeared to pop out of a children's storybook. Over the next few months, I walked through the world like a child; anew. I had come undone and through my connection to Straif, I began to weave a new life, a new outlook and way of combining the Universal secrets into something even more magical, as part of the physical world.

I spent hours walking along the hedgerows, watching as the Primroses gave way to the Campion and the Cornflower. Delicate orchids occasionally poked through patches of Wild Pea and the Blackthorn burst into blossom; showing me that all was well. Every flower whispered secrets, so integral to our Earth and to who we are that that I would cry with joy. I walked through the grove, sharing silent moments with the Sanctuary Oak and my other friends there. I visited the Lord of Thorns and the Little Blackthorn, I danced and giggled with rabbits on the moor, who seemed unafraid of my presence – something that is unheard of for such timid creatures!

Each day, my ability to interact with the natural world around me at a vibrational level became crisper, easier to grasp and more internal to my physical being. These interactions were less 'clunky' than the usual routines of therapy practices; of triggering Essences and running through many physiological movements. The connection just appeared, though not as I had experienced it before – now it was all-encompassing, as if I were a part of the natural environment, as opposed to an observer.

I freely gave myself time to consider what had transpired over the recent months and what factors had led to me to leaving myself so vulnerable. It was not long before I realised how much I had wanted a change. Working so hard each day for the development new forms of therapy and simply coping with my teaching commitments were gradually meaning that I did not have time to take a walk or read a book. My health was suffering and I was not as joyous about my role as I once had been.

In many ways, I was given a choice – to quash rumours and take legal action, or to just let it happen so that I may find a little time to rest and recoup my passion. I opted for the latter and, at first, beat myself up for having to go through such a hideous time. Straif taught me that it was OK to let go and to take time out for myself for the first time in almost a decade of total commitment to my students and my work. Those who truly knew me and cared about me would be there when I was strong enough to return.

My reasons for explaining the power of Straif to you are these: no matter what you are going through; how awful or complicated or unbearable the situations you find yourself in are. If the world feels as though it has turned against you, nobody seems to care and you feel utterly isolated and depressed; turn to the Essence of Straif – it helped me when I could see absolutely no way out. It clarified and cleansed, not only regarding the issues I faced, but my entire outlook on life.

I can say this with total conviction, because I have ventured there. I have experienced those dark and lonely times, when the road ahead appears long and you wonder if you'll ever make it. When the clouds appear and the sun fades away. I know how it feels and I came back from that place, so that I could return with some real treasure – the map of 'get-back-from-the-brink'.

The miraculous thing is that Straif does not offer his Essence unless it is truly needed. He remains quiet and unseen; blending into the background, watching and waiting for those in strife to call for him. When his help is required, he answers the call with such tremendous compassion that the old life fades away and something wonderfully new takes its place.

# A Prickly Pair

Thorns appear to be yet another recurring theme in my adventures with Celtic Reiki; one that influenced my decisions as to which trees to connect to, harvest and include within the system. Sensible individuals with rounded, smooth and soft leaves tended to be higher up on my agenda. Jagged, prickly or in any way scimitar-wielding, on the whole, had me passing by quickly, no matter how much the plants called me. Thus, extensive Essences for many of the thorny plants arrived much later in the Celtic Reiki origination story.

When people think about tree hugging practices, many do so with a slight, rather disparaging smile. And this occurs upon the mental image of a person wrapping their arms around a grand, old oak tree – imagine their expression when visualising a person diving headlong into a dense patch of gorse bushes, all in the name of harvesting their Essence! And, in general, I can see why this might present a dispute in the sanity department. However, my main issue with the harvesting of pointy or 'sticky-outy' plants is not what people might think, as much as—it hurts when a sudden gust of wind whips the branches over your hands and arms!

If you have ever been thwacked by gorse bush or holly in high-winds, you will appreciate my hesitation in this endeavour. However, there came a time when I simply could not hold back the progress of these vital Essences and so, I took the plunge (and my chances) with a rather thorny beast I jovially refer to as 'Spike'.

Spike is a huge gorse that grows in the beautiful setting of Hengistbury Head in Dorset. The gorse of Dorset and the New Forest are spectacular, especially in the spring and summer, when in bloom. The vibrant, yellow flowers have a wonderful scent that fills the air with a smell, resembling coconut butter. Now, seeing as this is one of my favourite aromas, I had been known to spend quite a bit of time with my face stuck near the flower-laden branches of gorse bushes. And, consequently, have also spent quite a bit of time with flower-laden branches stuck in my face, literally.

Spike was not like other gorse bushes, he was different – he promised to go gently with me, especially as it was my first time with a gorse bush! I desperately wanted to work with the Onn Essence, having experienced the amazing vibrations of the Gorse Bach Flower Remedy, I knew that Onn would be an amazing augmentation to the Celtic Reiki methodology.

As I placed my hands into a small opening in the dense, vicious-looking branches, Spike seemed to widen the space as if to reassure me that I was not about to be impaled! The curious thing I remember most about the harvest was the blistery winds blowing across the estuary and how other gorse bushes, lining the road, were swaying quite noticeably. Spike remained perfectly still around my hands and arms, so it was not long before I relaxed into the processes at hand.

For twenty minutes I lost myself, listening to the soft, deep inner voice of Spike, as he narrated wonderful tales of beauty and creativity. He showed me pictures and sounds and every-so-often would immerse me in a cloud of heady scent, which I breathed in deeply with a feeling of expansion.

There was an integral sense of joy in the Onn Essence, which is unlike any other. Enchantment, tinged with a cleansing dynamic, which leaves one feeling blissful, yet somehow new. In the very first meeting, Spike washed away any doubts I had about harvesting plants with prickles. He was a true gentleman!

I have subsequently befriended many gorse bushes and whilst a very occasional mishap may occur (mainly due to me catching the gorse in question unawares) in the vast majority of the instances the Onn clan are an incredibly gentle species, who love singing and being beautiful – inside and out!

Now with this reassuring introduction into all things proficient in the gouge-department, let me tell you about one who was not as friendly as my friend Spike. A rather sneaky bush of the Muin Essence that I affectionately (?) named 'Miss Whiplash'!

Actually, I'm being a tad judgemental, because all trees and bushes have their own way of doing things; oak trees tend to want the harvester to perform some action on their behalf; hawthorns are partial to the sharing of vibrations; hazels like juicy gossip; blackberry bushes want blood (usually accompanied by pain; stabbing, stinging and then fiercely itchy irritation!)

I have so many fond, childhood memories of blackberry picking in the New Forest with my grandmother. She was a maker of the most wonderful pies and would bake fresh apple and blackberry pie at the end of a hard day of bramble picking. I am not quite sure if the picking of berries as a child had anything to do with the attitude of Miss Whiplash, even if most trees and plants are usually happy for you to pick their fruits; particularly if you promise to plant some of the seeds safely in the ground.

I encountered Miss Whiplash in the New Forest; one of my most treasured places. I was reminiscing about my childhood adventures; you know the sort… driving my mother slowly mad, not wanting to walk any further, when ponies attack…you get the picture! Then quite unexpectedly, something sharp and incredibly painful scraped across the back of my hand.

I snapped my head around behind me to find a rather giggly blackberry bush, around four feet high and quite dense. She laughed and asked if she had my attention!

"Yes!" I retorted, whilst rubbing my hand vigorously in an attempt to numb the soreness.

"Good!" She responded, appearing as one attempting to sound serious, while holding back laughter. "I want you to remove this thing from my branches!"

I stared at her for a brief moment, pondering over what she meant by this demand. After no clarification was forthcoming, I crouched down and looked into her dense and spiky tangle of branches. Sure enough, deep within her menacing-looking undergrowth, was a bright blue carrier bag that had obviously become lodged after a gust of wind had blown it there.

"I heard that you're nice." She started again. "So do be a darling and take it away!"

When one communicates with trees or other plants in the lost language, it is not a spoken conversation as such, nor do I believe that the tree 'talks'. I understand the communication to be a

# A Prickly Pair    145

translation of the vibrational fields, as interpreted by the unconscious mind. Thus, if Miss Whiplash could have verbalised her wishes, I am convinced that is the manner she would have.

After a minute or two, I made the decision to help and crouched down even further, extending my hand into the undergrowth and towards the carrier bag. Being quite a way in, I needed to lean forward somewhat and I really should add to this image the idea that I am not the most adept person when it comes to keeping one's balance! Creeping slowly forward in some strange, 'awkward crab' manoeuvre, I became aware of her branches gentle stroking my hair and thought, to myself "This is OK, she's like the gorse and is being placid."

At this point, if somebody had been observing me with a camera that could capture a continuous series of rapid shots, they would have certainly obtained several new yoga positions. It is amazing how, when falling headfirst into a bramble bush, one can still be aware that the instinct to grasp on to the nearest thing is probably not the best motivation in this instance. What also provides an interesting point to consider at this juncture is how one can create delicate little pincers with one fingers, whilst attempting to tenderly cling to a piece of branch without multiple layers of spiky thorns waiting to flay the skin off your hands!

Hence, in one of those slow-mo moments that seem to be habitual in my Celtic Reiki journey, I careered into the awaiting mesh of serration, looking like a rhino with muscle spasms.

What was even more amusing to any observer, with a camera or not, would have been the instantaneous bouncing back into the upright position, when repelled by the spring action of the branches, united with the body's automatic reaction to 'get away from the sharp things'. The fact that I brought half the bush and the blue carrier bag with me on the way up, could only add to the humour quotient!

As I untangled bits of bramble branch from my clothing and began to feel the sting of various cuts on the top half of my body, Miss Whiplash chuckled to herself. A short while later she calmed herself and asked if I would like to harvest her for inclusion into Celtic Reiki. While, exfoliation to the point of blood-letting is not a practice I would recommend to the would-be Celtic Reiki Master, I did conduct a hurried harvest of Miss Whiplash, encouraged to act quickly by the intermittent bouts of stifled amusement, emanating from her direction.

The Muin Essence is actually quite amazing, with a balance between loving joy of life and a defensive nature that can be used to extreme effect in assertion, the Bramble is both beauty and the beast in one!

So, next time you go a-blackberry-picking with carrier bags to collect your booty, please do remember to take them home with you again – just in case I am passing by at some later date. In fact, better still – please take Tupperware!

# It's Elemental, My Dear Watson!

The creation of the Elemental Essences came about as a way of expressing different aspects of the natural world. The energy of our planet and indeed, 'all energy' is completely interconnected. Thus our ability to comprehend and connect to energy requires definition for the conscious mind to function. We are unable to consciously comprehend the infinite nature of energy, if we push our boundaries only slightly, there tends to be a profuse dribbling of brains out of ears!

By defining 'these' vibrations of energy under 'this' label and 'those' as 'that' Essence, we allow ourselves a way of connecting to small, finite 'chunks' of energy. This does, however, tend to limit and confine the way we observe energy; this translates in some instances to the view we are separate from energy, or energy is limited in some way – remember that definition is limited, energy is not!

The formation of the Elemental Essences enabled Celtic Reiki Masters to define different aspects of an Essence for treatment, teaching, or other practices within the methodology. The sun, the air, water and the Earth all played a significant part in the foundation descriptions of each, individual Essence, though I wanted to create an Essence connected to the concept of 'space' and separation. This was not the separation of loneliness, but of meditative contemplation and neutrality – a place to sit and think and observe an Essence with a sense of disconnection. For, as we trigger and connect an Essence in Celtic Reiki, we are affected by it and to a certain extent, shift our own perspective to that of the Essence. The ability to sense an Essence without the automatic immersion within its vibrations, means that a Master can glean a more detailed idea of what the Essence achieves from their own perspective.

Thus, Bearn (Space) became the first of the five essences for Celtic Reiki, which encompass the elements of our world. Connecting us to different aspects of the Celtic Reiki Essences, so, for example, if a Master wishes to create a more grounded effect in their treatment, Pridd (Earth) Essence creates a greater physical connection. On the other hand, a lighter result calls for the use of Annal (Air) in treatments.

Space creates a void; a point where energy is non-reactive and therefore neutral. This creates the illusion of there being 'no energy' to our senses whenever Bearn is triggered. Nevertheless energy exists everywhere and so it is Bearn that simply halts our reaction with energy.

This tends to mean that Bearn Essence is the first choice when working with those who are experiencing massive reactions to energy or emotions. For instance, somebody may be dealing with huge, internal struggle. This can create drastic health issues as we attempt, at an unconscious level, to cleanse the foundation challenge. Bearn disconnects them from this internal conundrum, so they have time to recoup, recognise their issues and release them without exertion.

If, at any time, a client is connected to something they feel is harming or draining them, a

Master will direct the Bearn Essence at the source of damage (as opposed to the subject). This disconnects the client from their focus by making it neutral to them.

The Tan (Fire) Essence adds vibrancy to any treatment and creates vibrations with greater potency of force. Tan is magnificent at stimulating and energising any Celtic Reiki work, transforming treatments that could have a soporific effect into revitalising adventures, while still retaining their relaxing qualities. Now, because fire does burn wood, the actual Tree Essences can lose some of their individual characteristics in place of the energetic power, yet, depending on the circumstances, this can be more conducive than conducting a treatment which pushes a person too far from alertness and awareness.

A fascinating aspect of Tan is derived from the actual harvesting of the original Essence, which consisted of two sessions; one with fire and the other with sunlight. This dual nature to the essence means that one facet of Tan creates a distortion of Tree Essences, like music that is played very loudly. The other layer (sunlight) creates an inner-bursting of energy from the Tree Essence, rather akin to a tree on a summer's day; reaching upwards to the sky and singing with joy as it replenishes itself with golden rays of sun.

The water element is represented by the Dwr Essence, which offers a smoother flow of energy vibrations. This can be witnessed particularly clearly on emotional and cerebral levels, if resistance (in the form of emotional or mental trauma) prevents treatment. The fluidity of Dwr makes it a fantastic choice when performing treatments that envelop the person being treated. It simply washes through them, invigorating, yet cleansing and calming. Adding Dwr Essence to a treatment will enable a Master to create 'mood' and atmosphere in the subtle changes it makes to the other Tree Essences used. Additionally, in contrast to the powerful qualities of Fire, the Dwr Essence refines the details within tree vibrations, softening and refining them.

I so enjoy harvesting Celtic Reiki Essences; the energy, the healing and empowering effects of the harvest, as well as the stories I discover along the way! Dwr was a particular pleasure to create, as I was able to spend time around natural sources of water. Dipping my fingers into babbling brooks, fast-flowing streams, still and enigmatic lakes and dramatic waterfalls, were all part of this beautiful essence. The most amazing thing about the harvesting process (in addition to the fact I actually managed to survive without massive injury!) was how different each facet of the process feels. From the gentle tingling of a tiny stream to the overwhelming buzz of a mountainous river, which seems to vibrate through the whole body from the feet upwards, every new feature to the Dwr Essence changes it in vast ways. Thus Dwr is one of the most fluid and adaptable essences – and so it should be!

The Essence of the Air: Annal lifts all connections to the Celtic Reiki vibrations offering a lighter and expansive feel to the treatment. Valuable for people who are tense, closed, physically orientated to the point of being stuck, those who are too focussed on 'stuff' or who are having difficulty in being without doing – i.e.: cannot mediate, relax, do nothing and just 'be'. Annal is like applying a treatment with a feather, it is always soft and gentle, embracing as opposed to cleansing (though it can also be used as the wind to clear limitations, stagnation and nurture one into movement).

I was born under the astrological sign of Libra (with Aquarius rising!) and have always tended toward the air and the ethereal. The sensation of dancing with zephyrs or the exhilaration of standing my ground in the path of howling gales that threatened to carry me off, were both equally as enjoyable for me.

The intangible, capricious nature of air is encapsulated in the Annal Essence, similar in many ways to Dwr. The inspirational lesson for me with Annal was how a Celtic Reiki practice can be adapted and changed, depending on the manner in which different Essences interact. Trees whisper in a soft breeze, bend in violent storms, they can be clear in shape and form on a perfectly still day and amorphous and constantly shifting when the winds tease their branches.

The various harvests of mountains, hills, wide fields and sandy deserts all comprise elements of the Pridd (Earth) Essence. Pridd grounds the connection to the treatment, bringing it more into the physical, creating deeper clearings and more integral change. Using Pridd enables a very material and physical connection for the Master, bringing the effects of each Tree Vibration to earth. Here a combination of essences can produce greater degree of detoxification and a much greater healing effect or faster and more direct manifestation of goals.

On every occasion I work with Pridd or one of the other Celtic Reiki Essences, I feel an integral sense of thanks and privilege for the adventures I have had. Every single harvest and essence is a memory; a personal, vivid and heartfelt reverie of a life lived as a celebration of the natural world and in particular our tree friends. The moments I have spent in connection to the plants, trees, mountains, oceans and the stars is like a photograph, stored deep within me; just waiting to trigger another story. Some are profound and deeply emotional, others funny, causing me to chuckle, and then there are those that leave me still, ponderous and quiet.

Being blessed with Celtic Reiki has given me so much over the years, from experience to wisdom to happiness. Yet, one thing that I have also been shown is how to be a better person; how to transcend the everyday 'stuff' that appears to be so important and yet is nothing when compared with the gigantic, 'bigger picture'.

The times I experience a transcendence of the mundane most clearly are when in connection to the mighty 'Mor' Essence – the Ocean. From the Atlantic, Indian and Pacific Oceans to the Arctic, the Mediterranean and the Red Seas, the huge expanse of ocean across our world, always fills me with awe.

As the original Master Essence of the first version of Celtic Reiki I taught, I have always shared a close affinity with the sea. I have played in the sea for many a long hour, swimming with whales and fishes, drifting peacefully on the surface and diving amongst coral reefs. No matter what activity I am partaking of, when it comes to the ocean, I am always filed with the sense that the sea is a sentient creature. Sometimes playful or mischievous, sometimes powerful and strong, and sometimes deadly, the deep hides the answers to many mysteries and is a very fickle creature. However, I have always had a deep sense of benevolence when in contact with the sea. There are times when I have known that I can relax, for I am safe in her arms. There are other times when she says, "stay away!" and I know to obey. He has listened when I've told him my troubles, and offers his essence freely.

There is an amazing life force about the sea that gives it such character and personality, though it changes from place to place. This is instilled in the many facets of the Mor Essence, one of Celtic Reiki's most multi-faceted essences, for it can be triggered as an overall essence, or in part by naming the different seas and oceans from which it is created. The extent of Mor's vibrations traverses the globe and transcends human borders; making Mor all encompassing and nurturing of all cultures, races and beliefs.

The sea holds the truth – the inner depths of knowledge and wisdom. We spend much of our lives on the surface of a rough ocean, letting life take us on its waves and seeming to have no say in the direction we want to head in. The Mor Essence enables us to sink down into the still depths of the sea where we can travel through life with ease and calmness.

Mor is about unknown wisdom and everything that a person can know. It compels us to learn spiritually, cerebrally, emotionally and physically. It guides and shows us sacred places and themes that we never even knew existed.

# The Bush That Burned

As the range of Celtic Reiki Essences expanded beyond that of the Celtic Trees (Trees thought to be held sacred by the Celts), to include other species of trees, the actual practise of Celtic Reiki seemed to become more pertinent to modern challenges and issues. It was as if the Celts had the answers they needed in the trees of their forests and woodland. We however have grown to the point where we need other types of Essences to deal with the complex and rather non-Celtic issues of our lives.

I had already developed connections to trees, such as Copper Beech and Eucalyptus when working with the therapy of Lemuria, yet had kept these separate from Celtic Reiki practise. My reasons for this were mainly centred around the idea of Celtic Reiki being complete with the traditional trees, however I was now realising that Celtic Reiki was about our tree friends, and not as much about the Celts or Reiki as I had once believed.

I therefore set about working with every variety of tree that wanted inclusion, from Cedar to Chestnut, Sequoia to Sycamore. I worked with the Elm, who is actually a Celtic Tree (Ailim), but had been relegated in the modern perspective of Celtic philosophy because of Dutch Elm Disease. Elemental Essences became part of the system, adding an even richer dimension to treatments and more recently, plants such as Fern, Bluebell and Rhododendron played their part in the creation of the most advanced form of Celtic Reiki. Add to this the Elven Essences and we now have a wonderfully plentiful modality of energy art.

Yet, still something was missing; an elusive piece of the overall symmetry that I could not define, yet knew was needed. Of course, I had actually comprehended at this juncture that Celtic Reiki will never be complete – it is an open-ended and constantly evolving creature that evolves with every new Master and each new perspective that hones an Essence. Still, the question of that absent chunk played on my mind.

Celtic Reiki had naturally discovered, over the years, its own unique balance of Essences – the Celtic Tree Essences and Mistletoe Master Essence, the Elemental Essences with Ocean Master Essence and the Elven Essences with Cernunnos Master Essence, however the Non-Celtic Tree Essences formed a seemingly random catalogue of vibrations; a conglomeration of different trees and plants, without direction or orientation. If the Celtic Essences were like naturally growing woodland, the Non-Celtic Essences were akin to a garden centre! As a group, they needed a Master Essence, some form of order and aesthetic.

The answer I had been searching for came on a trip to Egypt and the Sinai Peninsula and it was a metaphor that even I could not have expected! For just as a man called Moses had witnessed a fire laden tree thousands of years prior to my arrival, I too was about to have a run in with the very same bush! What I did not expect was the fire of a very different kind!

On the same trip, I had been able to work with several trees, including the Acacia, which is a beautiful fellow and an amazing testament to the ability for life to survive in the most inhospitable of places. I met and worked with several huge olive trees in the gardens of St. Catherine's Monastery and even some of the giant Sinai Cedars that are renowned around the world.

I walked amongst the ancient pomegranate and fig trees, soaking up the ambience of this magical place. One of the most wonderful aspects of this experience was how the Egyptian trees adapted so easily to the concept of Celtic Reiki, eagerly partaking in the harvest experience. And why wouldn't they; the natural world philosophies of the Celts are universal at a base level.

Exploring the monastery and the grounds was a chaotic and pleasantly dizzying experience of different cultures, beliefs and people. The most exciting feature of the trip was a chance to see the legendary Burning Bush; the very bush, written about in the Bible; portending Moses' experience on Mount Sinai and the giving of the Ten Commandments.

I was half-expecting to come across a miniature bush or tiny Acacia tree and there was even a part of me that thought there might be flames!! The huge, prickly bush that sprawled outwards from a high wall, was not what I presumed to find as I turned a corner of the monastery. The assembly of people milling around under the canopy of the bush, touching, pulling, or even ripping off pieces of twig was also quite a surprise too. I wasn't prepared for such disrespectful practices and even though I'm not a follower of any organised religion, the sheer lack of regard for this sacred tree was quite extraordinary.

I walked forward towards the tree and suddenly an all-encompassing pain ripped through my body. Sharp and burning, my entire body was rapt by muscular paralysis for an instant, followed by deep, internal shaking with the intensity of the sensation.

Standing completely still for a while, my head swimming from the unexpected wave of burning, the only words that I could think of were, "I've been smote!"

Finally, God has managed to catch up with me and dealt out a swift bout of smiting, as (I'm led to believe) is His prerogative! My second thought concerned cystitis, but we won't go into that here.

My third thought was an overwhelming sense of love and peace. It was as if the crowd slipped away and just left the bush and I connected by a deep benevolence. There were no words, no inner voice, no imagery or any form of sound. It was not unconsciousness or silence, just a calming of the outside world – there, although far away from me.

The ground seemed to come up to meet me, even though I was still standing perfectly upright. Swimming in this amazing sensation that completely filled my body, yet was beyond the physical, I stumbled towards the bush and lifted my arm to touch the branches. I felt warmed by some internal energy that rippled through me, dancing and singing to a rapturous melody that was beyond my comprehension.

What I can best describe as an in-body music that was not of sound, or even vibration, but of bodily sensation. Senses, thoughts, movement all colliding into a heady and disorientating experience that, looking back, seems fragmented and vague. It could be assumed that I would recollect something so utterly amazing; however, it was so 'not of the physical realm' that it seems impossible to vividly describe or even recall in the solid world.

The Essence of that extraordinary experience, even now evokes identical, physical sensations, the same emotion and complete cerebral incapacity. The vibrations are like many voices, all singing together in harmony; but not voices; perspectives. Maybe this is a chorus of angels, or a spiritual gathering of all the sacred trees that have ever lived, perhaps, simply of all trees? It could be a greatly expanded vibration of energy, or a mind-blowing satori. Whatever happened on that day at St Catherine's Monastery, I know that the Burning Bush Essence is a powerful and phenomenal healer and source of spiritual awakening. I have not been the same since and I doubt I can ever go back to the person I was before I was introduced to this most mystical of trees.

For that very first moment of connection to the Burning Bush, I knew I had discovered the Master Essence of the non-Celtic Trees. A potent reminder of compassion and deep rooted love for all trees, regardless of their species, where they grow, or what their perspective may be. If humankind could be united by these vibrations, this powerful energy as it has done for the Essences of Celtic Reiki practice, our global society, various nations and different communities would all surely be much more harmonious. And this was the very essence of the Burning Bush – to create a world of bliss for all living things, where the old notions of hatred, suffering, and cruelty no longer acquire sanctuary in the hearts and minds of people; where all life is held as sacrosanct, whether it is that of a human being, or the smallest of creatures, or a humble tree. And when we need to take life in order to sustain our own lives, we do so with respect and love and immense gratitude for the sacrifice that is being made. For when we cherish the gifts we have been given and hold all life in high esteem, we will truly know what it is to be human.

We are custodians of this planet and, just as the trees have done for millions of years before us; it is our duty to honour the Earth. We are all invited to create even more beauty for every form of life that lives here and those to come after us. Our legacy can be so much greater than we are establishing at moment, it can ensure happiness and health and bliss for all, during the fleeting moments of time that we are here.

These are the precious lessons of the Burning Bush and my hopes for the future.

# Farewell to Old Friends

Since I first embarked on my adventures in Celtic Reiki practice and beyond, I have connected to some of the most profound experiences imaginable – or in most cases unimaginable! On several occasions, these have consisted of the most joyous events and wondrous emotions, and at other times, moments of intense sadness. Through all of these experiences, my tree friends have been beside me, in physicality or in spirit. They have enriched my life beyond measure and I hope that in some way, I have managed to reciprocate this kindness for them.

So, before I complete this collection of reminiscences from my Celtic Reiki journey, I would like to share one last memory of those I have loved and lost. These friends are no longer with us in the physical world, yet remain very much alive through memories, thoughts and the celebration of their achievements – though seemingly small and insignificant to some, each tree and plant that I have met has contributed immense value to the world. This value is recognised here, with the hope that it inspires you to take the small and simple steps, which can lead you to make the world a better place; a wiser and happier place.

For when you have wandered around garden centres and shops, listening to the heart-wrenching cries of pot-bound trees that have not been watered for days and are burning in the sunlight; Once you have felt the agony of hedgerow trees and bushes, mangled haphazardly by cruel flaying machines; when you witness mindless acts of vandalism against trees; if you are surrounded by these experiences, simply because you have taken the time to notice them—you will probably feel as I do: that our friends, these life-giving, beautiful custodians need us. And I do not believe this is a case for *"thou shalt not..."*, because that approach rarely works. If we can instil within people, just how precious trees are, how valuable they are to all ground-dwelling life on Earth, and their important role in our continuation as a species, maybe then we will see changes.

I can recall one bright, spring day while visiting the Lord of Thorns, I immediately noticed that she seemed particularly sad. If she had eyes, I would have said they were gazing wistfully across the moor, in the direction of Plymouth. As I approached, she roused from her reverie and became much happier. When I asked what troubled her, she did not reply for the longest while. I persisted until she told me that, on occasion, she felt a pang of loneliness. In this rather sparse corner of Cornwall, trees need to be incredibly hardy against the fierce winds that howl across the wide moorland. Thus, very few survived, especially here, on the high hill where the Lord dwelt, guardian to her ancient, little field.

I decided to find a friend for the Lord, a little companion to plant nearby, who would act as company for her and a reminder that she was loved very much, by at least one human! So I began my quest to find a friend and was not searching long, before I came upon a little Ivy, who was very eager to grow beside the Lord.

For several months I nurtured the imaginative named, 'Little Ivy' with treatments and vibrational remedies, gradually preparing him for the harsh environment of the moor. For several months, I watched him grow, his tiny branches growing longer and stronger, uncurling away from the main growth of his body and unfurling minute green and yellow leaves. These slowly developed into rich foliage, robust against the cold and wind; he was ready.

I brought Little Ivy to the Lord, who was overjoyed, as I presented him to her. It was quite phenomenal to sense such a large and regal tree become a giggling mess, over such a small plant. Yet, despite appearances, he was not a small plant; he was a brave and caring individual. Little Ivy was prepared to leave the opportunity of a sheltered spot, safe in a garden to be planted in a rather hostile and bleak place. He did this freely, for the kindness of ensuring another was a little less lonely.

I planted him beside the Lord, with adequate space between them, so he would get a great deal of sunlight, though sufficiently close to guarantee some shelter from the worst of the wind. The two appeared to be very happy as I left them there in the twilight; the majestic holly tree and the impish ivy.

For several weeks they watched over the field together, contented and delighted with the other's company. Little Ivy's growth was certainly stunted by the transition to the harsher conditions, but still he seemed chirpy. He reminded me a boisterous young boy, carrying out a task he was obviously not sure about, but determined nonetheless to complete what he had set out to do.

I would bring fertilizer with me several times a week and spend time with the pair, giving Little Ivy the best start I could in his new home. The Lord was very different after she had gained her new companion; no more did I sense her pensive and contemplative demeanours. She had a friend by her side, to support her in her adopted duty as a guardian to this place. What is more, she knew that somebody would go to great lengths to ensure her bliss and I get the impression that was the greatest gift of all.

Two months after Little Ivy was planted on the moor, he was gone. I was visiting the Lord and Ivy as usual and I knew something was afoot as I approached her. She was tangibly distraught with vibrations, akin to static and that could be felt quite a way off.

When I reached her, I looked for Little Ivy, but all that remained was a couple of thin twigs, poking through the ground and one tint leaf. His leaves had been taken by a passing sheep and with only one remaining; he would probably not survive much longer on the moor. The Lord was furious and mourning her loss – it was so pitiful that I said I would take Ivy back with me and nurse him to health. I dug up his meagre frame and did as I had promised.

Once back inside, Little Ivy started to recover over the next few days, with visible growth on the twig with the remaining leaf and two new buds. Though, not even a week later he died during the night. I know that trees do suffer from shock, nevertheless they usually survive it. Whether it was the shock that killed Ivy, or just that he had lost so much of his foliage, I cannot say. Maybe it was the loss of the Lord that spurred Little Ivy to make the choice to die. Whatever the reasons, the Lord was left bereft without his company and I shall never forget this precocious little plant.

Despite the loss of Little Ivy, he does live on through the Gort Essence and this is the amazing aspect of the Celtic Reiki Essences. For they seem to preserve the memory of our tree friends, even after physical death. Energy is eternal; it exists beyond the confines of space and time and therefore, exists at every point of space and time. Whenever the energy of an Essence is used, we are making a connection to the source trees and plants themselves. In many way these are not memories of those now gone, they are bridges back through time to connect, once again, to those we love.

A while after the loss of Little Ivy, I discovered Little Yew tree, who wanted to be another companion for the Lord. At the time I was planting yew trees in various areas to increase the population of yews across the UK and the two needs appeared to be resolved by the planting of Little Yew, just a little way away from where Little Ivy had been. The Lord had never truly recovered from her loss of her companion and I felt I had to do something to help. My desire to help my holly friend was as lasting as my inability to pick inventive names for my tree friends! Therefore, with renewed optimism and a slightly happier Lord, Little Yew settled into his new home.

A week later, upon visiting the Lord, I noticed something rather strange nearby. It was mid-Autumn at this point and in the copper-tinged bracken, near the yew tree was an elongated orb of deep blue light. I had never witnessed anything quite like it and watched fascinated as the light hovered only a few feet away from me.

I enquired of the Lord what this peculiar occurrence was and received the simple reply that this was 'royalty'.  As I continued to observe the orb, it appeared to be looking at me in return. We gazed at each other for a number of minutes and then the light moved towards Little Yew. I watched in awe as the light settled over the tiny tree and seemed to 'merge' with him. It was then I realised this must be some form of dryad (tree spirit).

I was elated to think that Little Yew was connected with such an auspicious dryad. Maybe this was a sign of the yew tree's chances of surviving the trials of the moor. Yet, sadly it was not to be, as the next summer he too was gone. Having lost much of his foliage, through the harsh conditions, he seemed to just give up.

Over many weeks he faded and I came to realise that he and the Lord had taken time to contemplate the future. For as he slowly died, she did not seem as lost as she had previously. Maybe all they needed was a bit of time to say their goodbyes. I now know that most trees tend to perceive death as part of a cycle and accept it much more readily than we do. The Lord's reaction to the death of Little Yew was far less drastic than that of the Little Ivy, not because she cared any less, but down to the way of departure. With time to prepare, there was very little grief – the suddenness of her ivy friend's death was the root of her agony, not the fact that he died.

From this realisation, I learnt a valuable lesson. In life we never know what is to come, no matter how intuitive or psychic we may believe ourselves to be. No matter what methods we use or how we try to control the flow of our perception, there will be times when we fail to perceive loss or the end of a cycle. Hence, if we always act in a manner that saturates every situation with love and compassion, regardless of what transpires, we will have no regrets or need to look back and say, "why didn't I act in another way?"

Death is not only an ending, it is a beginning also. We are not destined to stay still, as so many people attempt to do, repeating old ways and stagnating in the process. For change and cycles are integral aspects of living. When we regard change as transformation and welcome it when it comes, we see death in a very different light. Life becomes about living every moment to the absolute full. By living in the moment, knowing that things will be different one day, we develop the tendency to love without condition. This is because as we remember each moment is finite, we feel compelled to inject energy into each quantifiable moment.

As our source continues to dance in the limited world of solid matter (sunlight and leaves), we evoke the very life purpose we came here to fulfil: to remember who we truly are! In the confines of the physical world, we are often distracted by the illusion, thus forgetting our true nature. However, when we recognise that time, with all its limits and scarcity, can overflow with the infinite love and joy of source; limitations become insignificant and the time we have is revealed to be a constantly shifting adventure through the beauty of the Earth.

We play like children amongst the trees of the forest and the grove, telling each other stories about our quests and experiences. We frolic until there are holes in our socks and wisdom in our hearts and our eyes feel heavy. We giggle and squeal for joy until bedtime, when it is time to sleep, to remember a day filled with fun just once more and then to dream new adventures in new, undiscovered lands.

# The Essences of Celtic Reiki

Every Essence that exists as part of the overall Celtic Reiki methodology is not merely a collection of energy vibrations; it is the shared perspectives of the trees that aided us in its creation. Each Essence consists of many stories and experiences, garnered over time by the trees, and deciphered by all the Celtic Reiki Masters who contributed to the harvesting.

The Essences are a lost language, perhaps used by our ancestors to live in harmony with the natural world, but now rare in the cities of the Western world. They are being rediscovered at a period of vast human evolution; for we are partaking in a major paradigm shift of spiritual re-awakening. To cope with the huge changes that are occurring, we are re-learning how to live as custodians of our natural world, not controllers and pillagers of it.

As we discover how to communicate with the trees, the wind and the oceans, we take our immense advances in technology and knowledge and use them to care for and nurture our Earth. For the Celts made mistakes and had cultural rituals that were at best misguided. We can, if we want to, combine the best aspects of both eras to form something new, something wonderful, something that belongs to each of us and all of us; tree, human, and all livings things.

## Ailim – A – (Arl-m)

### The Fir, The Spruce, The Conifer, The Pine
### (Traditionally, The Elm)

Ailim is of the Silver Fir, the Pine, the Spruce and the Conifer – he helps to clarify vision and to see the way forward (the horizon). Ailim breaks down barriers to the lessons learnt over our life-time; increasing wisdom from the past, increasing the connection to Celtic Wisdom and binding this to our consciousness, thus solving current issues in a person's life. The essence is particularly useful in looking to the very distant future, in areas such as life goals or life's work and helps integrate a person with their purpose. It can also connect the user to their Celtic ancestry if appropriate.

**Physical**: Of particular use on the mucus membrane and for clearing the nasal and respiratory tracts. Also has been seen to be very effective on any condition of the bladder and urinary tract.

**Emotional/Mental**: Lack of vision – cannot see a worthwhile future. Ailim is excellent for those who are unaware of or deny their qualities and achievements. Guilt and self-reproach are other areas where Ailim can be of use. Fear and loss, especially loss of one's home (being uprooted or cut off from one's roots). For the explorer, the nomad and the migrant, Ailim gives comfort and creates a sense of home, wherever you are.

**Spiritual**: Spiritual Vision: a finding of a life path and awakening of psychic/intuitive abilities. For spiritual development and a widening of perspective on spiritual matters.

## *The Message of Ailim*

I help those who are lost and cannot find their way in the darkness – I am sight, I am vision, I am home. For those who have been hurt in terrible, sometimes near fatal ways I can bring peace and understanding to what cannot be understood. For those who have lost their homes or who have been forced to leave their countries and homelands, I offer sanctuary and the ability to live in new places and circumstances.

I can be the comfort needed wherever there is death and destruction. In war, I offer peace, and in heartache I offer healing. For those who have strived for many years on paths that have led them to dead ends or perceived failure, I suggest new perspectives and alternative ways forward.

I offer healing to the sick in all physical disease, pain and loss – especially where something has been lost such as a limb or after major surgery to remove diseased aspects of the body. I have an affinity with children who are unwell and suffering in physical and emotional pain; including those who have been so ill in their short life that it will affect them into adulthood or may even take them prematurely. I soothe those who have lost one or more of their parents and those who have suffered great trauma as children. I heal the pain inflicted by humankind on its fellows and the abuse that is done by one individual to another – both male and female.

I support those who have been attacked or raped, whether they are male or female and regardless of the gender of the abuser. I create strength and complete reconciliation where there is 'violation'.

I see all and I can guide you to a place where you are healed and completely loved. Even when you can see no path, no way forward, no hope, I am there standing above all others – so look to the horizon and see the tall, wise Spruce tree that stands proud and defiant against all pain and abuse: that is me and I am Ailim.

## Onn – O – (On)

### The Gorse

The Gorse creates a gathering of inner strength to help those who feel weak or unable to cope, filling them with renewed vigour; tapping into their own source of power and joy so that it empowers them in the future.

Gorse is a remarkable creature, for he possesses such fierce and prevalent thorns and yet is capable of such beauty. Onn seems to mirror so many people in our world, for his need to assert himself has created the thorns that drive many away, yet he proclaims his need for love with the beautiful flowers that shine like gold on a summer's day, filling the air with the sweet scent.

He says, "Come gaze upon my beauty, breathe in my heavenly scent, and touch me softly, but do not get too close as I will hurt you!"

In actual fact, the Gorse is not nearly as formidable as he may appear upon first inspection, for although he does have a barrage of thorns; he is a very gentle tree. I have reached out to touch Gorse plants during howling gales and yet they seem to stop their thrashing at the place where you touch them, almost as if they hold strong against the wind, so as not to cause you harm.

Gorse offers protection to much of the local wildlife, providing shelter in places that are often inhospitable or prone to extreme weather. The beautiful yellow flowers offer abundant nectar to the insects and carpet hills, valleys and moors with such vibrant beauty as to take ones breath away.

Onn works with the building of inner strength to help those who feel weak or unable to cope with renewed vigour; tapping them into their own source of strength and joy so that it lasts and empowers them in the future.

The Celts are believed to have viewed the Onn vibration as being a very innovative essence, used to stimulate the creative juices, nurture new ways of thinking, develop artistic ability and otherwise push the personal evolutionary process forward. The beautiful vibrations of Onn sparkle with colour and light, awakening the senses and giving a heightened perception of the world, enabling us to experience our lives through many different sensory experiences, as opposed to the five senses that are usually restricted in use.

Onn provides colour to those who only see in black and white, allowing them to experience the joy of coming from a monochrome world to one of brilliant Technicolor. The vibration of Onn is also wonderful at producing a balanced view of the black and the white for those who only want the colourful aspects of life. For instance, when dealing with people who sacrifice their spiritual journey or life path for the sake of hedonism, physical pleasure, materialism, addiction, etc. Onn reminds us that the black and the white are there to protect us from our human nature and ourselves.

**Physical**: Help for those facing physical death. Works well in alleviating the symptoms of depression and side-effects of hormone imbalances.

**Emotional/Mental**: Helps people to come to terms with the emotional effects of terminal illness and a facing up to death of the physical. Brings out the creative spirit and helps artist/performers connect to their own spark of inspiration. Onn assists with the gathering of inner strength to help those who feel weak or unable to cope. By providing us with renewed vigour, the Gorse taps us into our own source of strength and joy.

**Spiritual**: Restores faith for those who feel lost or have suffered some terrible trauma. Restores belief in the benevolence of source, life, and humankind.

## *Ur – U – (Oo-r)*

### *The Heather*

The Heather has been revered for centuries, particular the 'lucky' white heather that is so popular that it is now starting to disappear from the wild due to collection from those who wish to make use of its auspicious vibrations. A greater understanding of the energetic nature of plants and trees offers us the wisdom that you do not need to uproot or harvest the physical being in order to work with the energy it possesses.

The 'luck' vibration of Ur assists us in the manifestation of our heaven on earth, as we strive towards a better life for all living things. Whether you believe in the random nature of luck as a concept or see luck as being an expression of being in 'flow', Ur will help you to realise your goals and bring the opportunities and necessary situations towards you.

By connecting us to the Earth and the natural world, Ur enables us to see our goal from a higher perspective. The essence also helps us to seek out the deva and other forms of woodland entity who can guide us on the right way forward. This strengthening of connections to our unseen realms enables us to work with nature in an intuitive way, as opposed to analysing what we need to do. We thus we dissolve the barriers that we encounter and start to work with energy in a more integral way.

Excellent in manifestation and healing alike, Ur helps us to perceive the world in a very different way, whether it be helping us to attract prosperity, diluting our limiting beliefs towards money, discovering inner peace, calming the world around us, healing the diseased or healing the diseases within us.

The Ur essence was given to us by many different heather colonies that range in location across the British Isles, from Scotland, Wales, and various parts of England.

**Physical**: Diseases of the feet and ankles, especially fungal infections and issues with the soles of the feet, such as collapsed arches.

**Emotional/Mental**: Brings a sense of joy and prosperity into the heart and mind. Connects us to the true meaning of Wealth, not in a 'monetary' sense, but in the richness of life and happiness.

**Spiritual**: Tranquillity of the spirit and the sacred art of prophecy are both developed through use of Ur. Manifesting Heaven on Earth and connection to Deva of the woodland.

## *Eadha –E – (Ee-yur)*

## *The Poplar, The Aspen*

**Physical**: Excellent for the nail, hair and scalp, as well as strengthening the teeth and cleansing the skin.

**Emotional/Mental**: Eadha helps to overcome fear: fear of the future, of responsibilities that may seem overwhelming; of the path we take and of the individual gifts we bring to the world. Eadha shields from the burden of the road ahead, helping us to work through and cope with the issues that may otherwise have pulled us down. This essence is excellent at helping when the pressures of life get too much and a person fears that they cannot cope with the world around them.

**Spiritual**: Eadha strengthens our spiritual resolve and gives us the ability to shout down the terrors we have with a whisper.

## Ioho – I – (E-yo)

### The Yew

The Yew Tree is the Celtic symbol of eternal life, as the Yew can live for thousands of years, continually renewing itself in an eternal cycle; sending branches into the ground that root, forming a hollow trunk. Ioho, in my experience, triggers one of the strongest connections of all the essences and was the first to be made into a Celtic Tree Remedy and Celtic Vibrational Remedy.

Ioho also helps increase the potency of other essences when used in a treatment and will cement the essences together to make them more fluid while acting in synthesis with each other.

**Physical**: Ioho can help in cases of poisoning and also helps with diseases of the very young or the very old. It has long been associated with death and therefore can help the physical passing of a person. Works well on the kidney and liver area.

**Emotional/Mental**: Ioho can help a person to "come back from the dead" on an emotional/mental level and so is good for issues such as nervous breakdowns, SDI, severe mental trauma.

**Spiritual**: The beginning and the end, the light and the dark. Ioho has the ability to resurrect spiritual faith that is lost and to bring what is hidden to the light. Used to treat eternal cycles that cannot be broken, or to create cycles that help a person to move forward – for example, those who cannot stick to any task, who are unable to motivate themselves or seem to be on an eternal path that gets them nowhere. Excellent for people who always make the same mistakes and never seem to learn or still create the same cycles even after learning the errors of their actions. Ioho helps increase the potency of other essences when used in a treatment and will also help cement the essences used in a forest to make them more fluid while acting in synthesis with each other.

## *Beith – B – (Beh)*

## *The Birch*

Beith is of the Birch Tree and assists in the release of old ways, patterns, negative beliefs and reactions to energy. She clears the past to make way for the present and the future, helps us to work through issues that are holding us back, cleansing and letting go. She is also wonderful with helping to motivate at the start of a new venture. Often beginning something is the hardest thing to do—Beith will assist you in getting over any initial inertia in starting a new project.

Another side of Beith is that of forgiveness, helping us to forgive those who have hurt us in the past, she allows us to release any negative reactions to energy.

The Birch is the initiator; the tree of new beginnings and fresh starts and is very relevant in our ever-changing and evolving world. I have worked with many birch trees over the years and have had the opportunity to meet many different individuals of other birch species, such as a magnificent 'paper birch' whose vibration offers help and support to those who want to 'shed their old skin', or change in some integral way.

She also provides help for those with dry and flaky skin conditions such as psoriasis or eczema as well as helping ease the effects of flaky scalps and conditions of dryness/dehydration.

The ability to help those who are starting anew after changing or are coming to terms with a fresh start after some major transition or loss has brought the Beith vibration to a new level of effectiveness and created a greater integrity of the vibrations. This enables flexibility and rebirth as well as the processes of birth for the first time.

**Physical**: All skin conditions and muscular illness, or pain. It can also be used as an appetite suppressant for those who wish to lose weight.

**Emotional/Mental**: Creates a feeling of newness and renewed optimism for the future. Clears the past to wipe the slate clean and offer fresh approaches to old problems. Motivator and energiser.

**Spiritual**: Renews spiritual growth and enables us to accept new concepts with ease.

## Luis – L – (Lweesh)

## The Rowan

The Mountain Ash or Rowan was traditionally deemed to be a highly protective tree and this is revealed in the saying "No evil shall pass the shadow of the Rowan". The vibration of Rowan contains this ability and much more as, in addition to the energy assertion it provides; it also gives the ability to halt negative reactions to energy. Luis enables the discernment of whether you are being offered help or subjected to harmful intent.

The Rowan tree can survive in the most inhospitable places, breaking the murkiness with a vibrant display of red berries, attracting birds that shelter in its branches and fill the air with song. This is another aspect of the Luis Essence—when things are at their darkest, when all is doom and gloom, hope has drained away and there seems to be no way out—Luis will fill the air with a beautiful song, light up the shadows with vibrant colour and shelter us from the worse effects of the environment.

Work on the Luis Essence was started in 2001 and took two years to evolve. It began when I stumbled across a very poorly Rowan tree in a shop and decided to nurse it back to health. Having bought the tree I worked with Reiki to help the tree back to health – this process took a full turning of the seasons to complete. The happier Rowan now needed to be released from its bondage and I set about finding a suitable home.

It was in the Bodmin Moor Grove that I found an ideal spot – almost as if it had been waiting for the little Rowan. So on a cold autumn night, the Rowan was released to a new life and there it still stands amongst its peers and the ancient ones who can pass on their wisdom.

Since that time, Rowan is another genus of our tree friends that I have become most connected to over the years, with the individuals I met along the way being some of the most giving and beautifully natured creatures. In the Cornish Grove (being a place, predominantly populated by Rowan trees), it was only natural that I would meet many Rowans, yet I was unprepared for how many of these beautiful beings wanted to help with Celtic Reiki and generally.

This, in turn, has created one of the richest and most diverse of Celtic Reiki vibrations that are available to us. Whether connecting to the root essence of Luis or to the individual trees, we find so many loving and supportive elements to this aspect of energy that it is sometimes overwhelming in scope.

**Physical**: Boosts the immune system and helps with cold and flu symptom. Helps to ease tea and sugar addictions.

**Emotional/Mental**: Mental clarity and discernment are major aspects of this essence, along with the ability to assert emotionally and mentally, for example, from the likes of depression, despair and loneliness: when all hope has disappeared. Also stimulates creativity.

**Spiritual**: Spiritual protection and awakening.

## Fearn –F – (Fi-een)

### The Alder

It was in 2005 that I finally met an indigenous Alder, only ever having encountered cultivated trees of that species before. I was on a visit to Wales, where Celtic Reiki all began, when I passed through a Sacred Grove, whose energy was unmistakable akin to that of the Cornish grove. At the edge of this sacred place, a huge lake lapped the foothills of the Snowdonia Mountains and by the lake was a solitary Alder.

The tree was surrounded by stones that pulsed with energy, unlike anything I had felt before. It was obvious this tree was a guardian to something very powerful. Having treated the tree, lake and stones with homoeopathic remedies, I approached the Alder and explained about Celtic Reiki, before asking if I may use his vibration for Fearn. He said yes, but on the strict proviso that I only learn his vibration, taking nothing physical from this place.

Having agreed, I harvested the powerful energy of the keeper of secrets and still to this day I am unaware of what the guardian was asserting against. Thus the Fearn vibration was created and can be used on those who have the heavy spiritual 'burden' of secrets and the unknown – ancient and futuristic powers that they cannot share with others and thus are bound to silence.

It will also help those who are told the secrets of others and thus have a great power. It will help them to use their power wisely and be at ease with the responsibility they hold.

The Fearn Essence is also about remembrance and the passing of all things, it helps us to remember those we have lost and keep their memory alive within us. It also helps us to remember the things that we try to push aside, for they are too painful. By embracing what we fear most, we can connect to the energy and then repattern it to something that gives us strength – by avoiding our past and suppressing it, we give it more power and so it haunts us. If we learn to remember our past from a new perspective and one that helps us to grow, we can also discover our greatest gifts and potential.

Another use for Fearn is that of recapturing the memories of our past lives and those of our ancestral line, helping us to remove any negative karma that we have contained within us at a vibrational level. As we envelop ourselves in the lives that have gone before us, we can use the Celtic Reiki essences to treat those traumas and diseases that, extending forward in time from the past, hold us back in the here and now.

**Physical**: Issues of the lumber area, hips and pelvis. Joint pain, arthritis and rheumatism are all eased by the treatment with Fearn.

**Emotional/Mental**: Emotional force and strength of character, rather like the Duir Essence, yet more 'active' inasmuch as the Fearn Essence is more of a watchman than a gatekeeper. Thus, any situation that calls for a dynamic approach to assertiveness and action will be benefited by this essence.

**Spiritual**: Higher task and a sense of mission.

*Saille – S – (Sal-yur)*

*The Willow*

Saille is the Willow Tree and refers to the moon/lunar rhythms and as such has a very interesting nature. Firstly, the essence works in relation to the lunar cycle; therefore she is excellent at manifestation when the Moon is waxing (New to Full Moon) and treatment when the Moon is waning. Next of all, the willow has many interesting qualities, not only in treating others and manifestation techniques, but also when working with other natural energy.

Willow eases pain of all kinds, physical, emotional, psychological and spiritual, she also works well on skin conditions, any issue to do with the hair and issues of the heart. When used for fulfilment of wishes and dreams, Saille is best used in manifestations of the soul: to improve the ability to connect to higher levels, to work with guides; to help you clarify your life's work and discover your purpose. Saille is the manifestation tool for the spiritual that have travelled their path for a while and are ready for the next step. She will help you connect to work with Ley-lines and Stargates (Stone Circles) and connect you to the stars.

When I started to work with the trees of Celtic wisdom, Willow was one of the first that I harvested, with the help of a garden-bound Willow in London. She was an incredibly happy soul who enjoyed the sunlight and was very happy just 'being'. One thing that made me smile was her motherly nature, as she projected energy to all the other flowers, plants and trees in the garden to make sure that they were all happy too. When the Willow was happy, all around her were happy, especially the flowers, growing under her branches; they appeared to be the happiest bunch I have ever met!

Willows are often associated with grief – this is not due to the fact that they are unhappy, it is because they have long been located where there is much grief – so they can take it away...

A major development to the Saille vibration is the addition of Feather Willow, an ancient, ivy-covered willow in the Cornish grove. This tree is very interesting, not only for its wisdom, but also as it has neither male nor female qualities, but is androgynous, meaning that it is of a gender that we do not have in humankind, or the gender than can only be obtained by artificial means.

This means that Feather Willow can offer us a genderless perspective in issues of gender, such as communication difficulties between men and women, or problems with gender identity. For those who identify with a gender that is different to their birth gender or those who were born hermaphrodite, Saille works in creating understanding and truly positive identity.

Thus Saille is not about 'coming to terms with' or 'accepting' one's gender identity or gender issues – it is about revelation and true comprehension of our very individual and personal gender: creating equality and self-esteem within the individual that will be reflected outwards. The trees do not have sexual politics – they just are who they are and do what they do without judgement of others or themselves. These qualities can also be instilled, not only in people who have difficulty with their own gender or sexual identity, but in those who hate others because of gender or sexual preference.

Sexuality and gender-related issues affect us on physical, emotional and psychological levels but have no place in true spirituality, so cannot affect us there. However, as we grow up and develop, the second-hand limiting, dogmatic and prejudicial beliefs of our society and those individuals hungry for power, domination and control through blame, affect us and can create spiritual dilemmas. Saille can help us to view those of different gender and sexual identity as equals, with equal rights – this means that we accept all genders and sexualities within ourselves, so that we embrace our own sexual/gender identity completely.

Two other layers of the Saille Essence are derived from Willow trees that have been near death and yet recovered – one is a weeping willow, the other a corkscrew willow. Both of these trees nearly died, the corkscrew through lack of water and the weeping willow as it had been placed into a dormant state and packaged for sale in a convenience store. It never truly recovered from this, however the rootstock started to grow again, enabling the growth of a new tree to start.

Both of these small, yet beautiful individuals encompass the qualities of the original Saille Essence, yet here the meaning of survival after death and spiritual rebirth are apparent when we realise we can even overcome physical death to live on and whilst there is the smallest flicker of hope, we can make it through the pain.

**Physical**: Pain, such as headache and muscular ache/pain. Skin conditions, Hair loss, dandruff, etc. Heartburn, pain in the chest and heart. Physical illness caused by deep-rooted trauma.

**Emotional/Mental**: Emotional and Mental anguish. Trauma of all kinds. To sooth and calm the nerves and release bitterness/resentment from the heart area. Can also be used to make somebody laugh!

**Spiritual**: Use in powerful manifestations such as astral travel, vibrational bi-location, avatar qualities, ancient energy and communications, multidimensional work.

## Nuin – N – (Nee-arhn)

### The Ash

Since the creation of Celtic Reiki, I have worked with several Ash trees and encountered many fascinating individuals. One of the common themes that I have found with Ash is that, compared with the likes of Quert, Tinne or Saille, Nuin tends to lean more to the intellectual or cerebral aspects of energetic vibrations. Yet, unlike the other trees of knowledge, Nuin works in a very different way to Phagos, who enthuses knowledge like a child who has learnt something new and cannot wait to tell the world, or Huathe, who offers little chunks of information a piece at a time. Even Coll, the tree of knowledge, gathers her wisdom through 'gossiping' and hearsay – she is like the housekeeper who sees all and knows all the goings-on of the house, yet in the case of Hazel, she tells all – to everybody who will listen!

Nuin prefers to infer knowledge through example, creating action or reaction to his vibration that enables you to see the essence of the lesson played out before you. He is logical and practical, yet extremely benevolent and just a touch humorous in his style. If trees had jobs, he would be the college professor who is always one-step ahead of his students and has the ability to make you feel very big or very small.

Having liberated a beautiful Golden Ash to the sacred Grove, and being connected to various Ash trees of the forest and hedgerow, I have a real affinity with the Ash. In late 2003, I worked with many young Ash trees that bordered a road near where I lived at the time, connecting and 'chatting' to each. Only a few days later, every tree along the entire stretch of road was decimated by hedgerow flayers that were ensuring no branches interfered with the road – by hacking entire trees down. Needless to say I have worked with all the survivors and many of their stories and healing paths exist within the Nuin vibrations.

**Physical**: Balancing between left and right body. Health issues that affect one side of the body more than the other, or that change from one side to the other.

**Emotional/Mental**: Transmission of knowledge and the gathering of wisdom. Balance of mind and emotions.

**Spiritual**: The sacred nature of spiritual knowledge. Fluidity of perspective and the oral traditions of spirit wisdom. Expansion and growth

## *The Message of Nuin*

I am a path that grows straight ahead, yet when I develop branches, they form at the same place and stretch out in opposite directions. Thus, I offer a choice – to call upon our spiritual and higher aspects, to move towards the practical and logical path, or to continue on the path of balance. The answer may be different on each occasion, but all paths will eventually lead to the light.

I teach the inner and the outer, the very large in the very small – I am a paradox and an understanding that can only be felt and known, rather than understood. My essence can be called upon whenever you are dealing with many small issues or times of huge change. Where you encounter contrast and opposition, you may call upon me for guidance.

I also help on all levels, when dealing with the large and the small, such as the small in-growing toenail that affects the way you posture your entire body or the tiny worry that is blown out of proportion. I can help you on the path to enlightenment when the tiniest of blockages has completely halted your progress and I am always ready to help you work through the straw that breaks the camel's back!

Traditionally used as the connection during the beginning of a treatment or attunement, I initiate the end – for beginnings are always ending. I represent both the start of the treatment and the finish of dis-ease, the commencement of a new path towards the use of Celtic Reiki vibrations and the ending of old struggles and beliefs. My season is the first month of spring and while I represent the creation of new hopes and dreams for the coming year, I also encompass an end to the harsh months of winter.

Whenever you work with my vibration, observe what is not seen, what is not known and whilst you may not be able to truly grasp the hidden dynamics of my energy, be aware that in everything there is opposition and balance.

## Huathe – H – (Hoo-arth)

### The Hawthorn

Huathe is of the Hawthorn and his essence represents the force of cleansing and preparation. The clearing of thoughts, as opposed to physical actions. He is an excellent forerunner to the Beith essence; he clears the mind of negative thoughts and mental confusion, offering clarity. He gives patience and offers stillness and the ability to wait until the right time comes.

Can be used in conjunction with Ailim to calm and create a clear picture of the way ahead. Sometimes the way ahead can be obscured by too many thoughts; this will clear those thoughts, allowing Ailim to show the horizon.

Another use for the Hawthorn essence is in conception of life. It can be used to help increase fertility during the conception of a child, during the pregnancy and at the actual birth. Huathe will help smooth the process and create plain sailing for both mother and baby. The reverse is also appropriate, as this energy will help women through the menopause, lessening the harshest of the side effects.

Huathe was originally one of the least known Celtic Reiki essences, as I had only one occasion to work with a Hawthorn tree, rather precariously positioned on a mountain in Wales. As such, I had used Huathe very little in treatments. In a more recent turn of events, I came across several Hawthorn trees on Bodmin Moor and one particular tree called to me.

Whilst treating him with Reiki, this small, but wonderful looking fellow, asked me for some 'Sunlight'. Now, being midwinter, there had been very little sunshine and even on the more clement days, the sun had only been in the sky for a few hours. So I captured some sunlight in a bottle of water and on my next trip to the moor, sprinkled it around the Hawthorn and his nearby family. I instantly saw them brighten as the vibration of sunlight filtered through to them. The Hawthorn who had asked me to bring him the sun was very impressed and filled me with a blast of Huathe energy in gratitude for my efforts.

This was the first time I had attempted to give a tree sunlight, but since then, I have had many others in the local area make the same request. Hawthorns can gossip in the same way as Hazel trees!

Since that time, Hawthorn has become a tree genus that I have worked with extensively. It is not the easiest of species to work with and has taken its fair share of blood (which surprisingly is the way of Huathe). There is often a price to be paid, but the rewards are great! Huathe is unlike any other species of tree that I can mention. He is abrupt, to the point, acerbic and can be fickle – yet his wisdom and ability is second to none. He offers wisdom and magic from a very different perspective. In times of real need, this can be exactly what we need to get us through.

Hawthorn's ability to cleanse and prepare the way can often be misinterpreted as carelessness or may seem hurtful in its apparent lack of compassion, but Huathe does care – he just shows it in a very different way to other trees! Huathe enables us to realise that others do not appreciate us if we give ourselves freely – and when we give ourselves freely we assert to other levels of our being that we are not worth much. There must always be an exchange: a trade of information or of energy. To always give selflessly creates imbalance and that is never healthy.

Two other individuals in the Huathe Essence are the 'Old Hawthorne of Time' who gives us a very tree-oriented view of space and time and is very helpful to those who cannot grasp practical or physical concepts such as space (finding their way around) and time (can never get somewhere on time). Seeing an alternative perspective, albeit energetically, can really help us to come to terms with physical concepts that we usually only see from a human or society based viewpoint. There are many other ways of perceiving our world and not all of these take human form!

The other individual stands next to 'Sunshine Hawthorne' and is called the Clooty Hawthorne. Clooties were small pieces of cloth that were traditionally knotted around the branches of the Hawthorne tree when a person wanted to make a wish for something. Thus Clooty Hawthorne is an excellent choice when conducting a manifestation treatment or making a wish. Ask for his vibration especially when activating the Huathe Essence and he will help you to make your dreams come true – remember that there may be a price to be paid. This may take the form of losing some money/an object or maybe a small cut or bruise – you can always pre-empt this by returning a favour to Hawthorne through your own freewill and volition.

**Physical**: Can be used in conjunction with IVF. Pregnancy and Childbirth. Menopause. Works on the circulatory system and reduces blood pressure.

**Emotional/Mental**: Can help in matters of the heart: in both healing and releasing relationships. Will help to save a love that is dying – providing this is for the highest good. Can help those wishing to manifest a loving relationship or who wish to be parents.

**Spiritual**: Can help to nature unconditional, spiritual love for all things.

*Duir – D – (Doo-r)*

*The Oak*

Duir is of the Oak Tree and represents the month of May, the last month of spring and the end of the beginning. Duir is an excellent essence to employ near the completion of the first stages in a project. As the foundations of our work are complete, Duir will smooth over any rough edges and tie up any loose ends. Thus, he will help the transition to the next stage of a journey and is wonderful just before a full Moon.

Duir is the opener of doors and gateways. He lends those who have connected a great strength and knowledge of the mysteries contained in the universe. He protects and keeps the practitioner and client safe from any negative reactions to energy during the treatment or practice.

The initial gathering of Duir happened whilst conducting an Usui Reiki to an old Oak located in St James' Park, London. This mighty individual was very strong willed, but very benevolent towards his human visitors, feeling a great need to shelter people under his branches!

The Duir Essence still remains one of the strongest in Celtic Reiki – the influence of Sanctuary Oak is as strong over Duir as the Lord of Thorns is throughout Tinne. Yet with another grand Oak tree now added to the vibrations, we have an even more potent range of vibrations to Duir, with an added twist.

Wise Master Oak is located a few yards away from Sanctuary Oak and is one of the wise trees of the grove, in Cornwall. He is so benevolent and full of fascinating information, his energy is kind and loving, perhaps more so than any other Oak tree I have encountered.

Yes, I would say that all Oaks have love and compassion within them, yet their strength and assertion often shield us from experiencing this fully. With Wise Master Oak there is no hiding. He is like an old grandfather who likes to play with his grandchildren, telling them stories, offering wise advice and giving them the best and most loving start he can.

Wise Master Oak stands along with a group of young hazel trees that seem to be 'ladies in waiting' and who spend most of their time giggling and going all coy when I come along – especially if I have some organic fertiliser or homoeopathic remedies with me!

During the work with Unhewn Dolman Arch, I was working with the seeds of this most sacred Celtic Tree. Wise Master Oak was very eager, if a little nervous, to be introduced to the 'All Heal'. Some of the seeds were placed on his branches and wrapped in stocking to keep them safe from birds and insects. As the seeds were planted, Wise Oak changed; his vibrations became what I can only describe as 'regal'.

Oak trees containing Mistletoe were seen as the most sacred and honoured of trees by the Celts – there is something about the synthesis of Oak and Mistletoe that cannot be attained by any other energy. I witnessed this change occur as each seed was placed on one of Wise Oak's branches – how his energy develops and when the plants start to grow remains to be seen, yet it seems there are great things in store for the Duir vibration.

**Physical**: Back Pain, Diarrhoea, Food Poisoning and Fungal Infection. Addiction to Tea/Coffee.

**Emotional/Mental**: Lack of inner strength, weak and tossed about by life. Exceptional results to be found in those who are unable to put words or thoughts into action. People who hide the truth from others and themselves. Fear. Darkness.

**Spiritual**: Works well in manifestation and bringing the spiritual or energetic into physical reality. Offers a spiritual truth to the user and the receiver of the energy.

## Tinne – T – (Tin-nay)

### The Holly

The Holly is the protector of the Ogham. Unlike Luis, which protects from negative reactions to energy and influences, Tinne empowers an individual, enabling them to fight their own battles. The increased vigour and resilience produced by the Tinne energy allows people to assert themselves, especially when engaged in struggle where balance is required along with the need to 'keep it together'.

Traditionally seen as masculine or father energy, Holly can also be regarded as the maternal nurturer for, within the hard exterior of those spiny leaves, is a soft heart and over-powering love that is given completely unconditionally.

Hence, Tinne, acting as both father and mother, female and male, can show us an all-encompassing love that shows us how to love ourselves in a completely balanced way and from all perspectives.

The wisdom of Holly is unquestionable, automatically bringing to the light an answer to the most complex life question. There is often, however, a sacrifice to be made with Tinne energy, as it can be the case that, to find an answer, you may need to give something up. It is only afterwards that you realise you never needed it afterwards.

**Physical**: Pain relief. Speeds healing of broken bones. Sexual disease, or dysfunction.

**Emotional/Mental**: Calming, soothing and stress releasing. Holly can raise a fighting spirit or show the need for reconciliation or peace. Especially beneficial with deep-rooted anger, hate, jealousy and desire for revenge. Holly can help everybody to understand their sexuality, work with gender issues and integrate inner male/female aspects of their psyche.

**Spiritual**: Can provide sudden inspiration and intuitive knowledge. Gives an individual the ability to 'pluck answers out of the air'.

## Coll – C – (Cull)

### The Hazel

Coll is the Hazel, one of the most revered and valued trees in the age of the Celts. It was called the 'Tree of Knowledge' and the centre of all knowledge was believed to be contained in the Hazelnut, a very potent symbol for the Celts. The wood from the Hazel is said to have mystical powers and has long been sought after by those of the Wiccan faith for use in wands and staffs.

The Coll essence reflects this in her ability to enhance personal knowledge and awareness and, when used in a treatment, she can help to increase awareness in all aspects of the self. For example: it can put a person in touch with their body so that they will know what foods they need, how much physical activity they should partake in, what is harming their body, etc.

The Coll vibration can also put people in touch with other parts of themselves, such as their emotions, their higher self, their true self, etc.

The Hazel was also seen as the 'Emblem of Healing' and is therefore very therapeutic when used as a general 'tonic'. She will help increase your wisdom and inspiration in consultation environments and generally sensitise your intuitive abilities during a treatment.

Coll can also be used to increase the potency of all other essences, especially of Oir and the two work very well together.

Hazel is another example of a tree that I have come into contact with regularly and whilst Ioho, the

Yew, is the species with which I have the most resonance, Coll is a close second. I have worked with many Hazel trees across the UK, from Wales and Scotland, to Kent and Cornwall, and wherever I have travelled, I have always found the Hazels to be very giving and friendly folk.

One of my longest companions is a little corkscrew Hazel, who I rescued from slavery, as I did with Luis, the Rowan. Unlike Rowan, however, she has been much happier in captivity and shows no signs of wanting to leave. Thus she remains in a large pot with some scented flowers around her for company, until she decides otherwise!

Another aspect of the Hazel energy is that of the nut, which has also been added to the Reiki vibration of Coll. The nut in question was from a Cornish Hazel and the little seed travelled with me for many weeks as I learnt his energy. I then returned him to his rightful place: the ground.

What we sometimes do not understand about Hazels is how they get their information – of course the answer exists with the fact that the Hazels are the world's biggest gossips!

Hazel's art for hearsay is second to none as she chatters away constantly. The Hazel is never malicious or cruel in what she says, always laughing and keeping her dignity, but she has found that the best way to know all is to tell all!

The Coll Essence reflects this quality, as it offers us knowledge yet it is the wisdom of hearsay. In our factual world, we tend to trust books more than the Internet. If we see facts in an encyclopaedia, they are truer than the words of somebody we meet on the street and, if it is on the television—well, that is more factual than anything else! However we tend to attract in the information that we need at the time it is most relevant so, whether it is spoken or written in a book – the important thing is that it resonates.

It is better to believe something that fits perfectly with you and makes you happy, than to replace your beliefs with a fact that gives you no comfort and offers nothing but darkness – this is not deceiving oneself, for who actually has the right to say something is true and something is false? Everything, absolutely everything is perspective and hearsay, even science.

Coll will tell you exactly what you need to know, when you need to know it – so trust her. She may seem like a giggly schoolgirl on the surface, but she is a wise and loving woman, capable of the most profound wisdom and the most resonant knowledge.

**Physical**: Very good at enabling a person to look after their body better. Boost physical healing. Cigarette and Alcohol additions.

**Emotional/Mental**: Helps to calm and empower a person emotionally. Can lead a person to their life path and to recognise their positive and negative traits. Wisdom.

**Spiritual**: Increases spiritual knowledge and soul's journey. Good for use in self-treatment for all Energy Therapists.

*Quert – Q – (Kwert)*

*The Apple Tree*

Quert is the energy of love and beauty and can be used wherever there is a lack of both, whether this is a true lack or a perceived one. When treating those who feel unloved or who cannot see the beauty within them, Quert will fill their world with a harmony, peace and joy that is formed from the vibrant and essential energy of love and beauty.

Quert raises a person's self-esteem and enhances a well-rounded and realistic love of oneself, particularly useful in times of darkness or when feeling unappreciated by those around you.

The energy is that of gratitude and faith – of trusting in the processes of life and the wonder of the Universe and of being thankful for all that life has to offer. Especially valuable when we are focussed on the three-dimensional aspects of physical life and forget about the amazing gifts we receive each day but often overlook.

Physically, Quert works on the gastric system and the chest – excellent for any disease surrounding the heart or solar plexus chakras. It is therefore wonderful when used on asthma, bronchitis, pneumonia or upper digestive complaints, etc. Quert is an excellent cleanser and can help to clean the gut and the blood and is excellent when combating the symptoms of high-cholesterol.

The apple tree vibration also works well on mental and spiritual levels, helping a person to find and fulfil their destiny, to assist in the meeting of a soulmate or increase the love and passion within an ailing relationship. It also helps a person retain their generosity in times when things are tight and one might not feel like giving. Quert works wonderfully with Luis and Ruis.

This particular vibration returns us to the Cornish grove that has played such an integral part in the development of Celtic Reiki in the past year. A single crab apple tree stands in the Grove – it is right by the main road passing through this sacred place and yet is unseen and often missed by those passing. This friendly and loving individual completes the 'Sacred Tree' vibrations of the Celts and enhances the Koad energy also.

**Physical**: Chest and stomach issues. General cleansing qualities, especially of the colon and the blood.

**Emotional/Mental**: Beauty and love, especially Universal love or compassion. Quert helps us transition into the 'I Care' and 'Universal Care' stages of life, transcending selfishness and egocentric views of the world, in favour of a giving viewpoint.

**Spiritual**: Spiritual expansion and compassion. Powerful manifestation and energy magic abilities.

## *Muin – M – (Mhoown)*

### *The Blackberry*

Muin encompasses the vines, and in the case of the Celtic Reiki Muin Essence the Bramble, or Blackberry. This prickly, somewhat intimidating plant is one of the most prolific and hardy creatures in England, found commonly amongst the hedgerows that border our roads and lanes. This can be somewhat troublesome for the unwary hiker, yet they offer an abundant source of food for birds, animals and us blackberry lovers come September – the month of Muin.

Muin is balance and diplomacy, for it is equally defensive and yet enticing, for it offers a nasty cut to those who mistreat it, but such riches to those who act with care in its presence. The essence of Muin inherits this trait and gives us a range of vibrations unlike any other. This particular aspect of energy is used without intent and just projected at times you intuit during treatments, self-treatments or generally when you feel the need.

As you use the Muin vibration, it will act as a catalyst between your energetic fields and those around you. This means that when somebody has your best interests at heart, they will receive abundance, love and joy. As you meet and mingle with those who mean you no harm or will do right by you, Muin offers healing, balance and harmony.

However, when you encounter those who in some way want to hurt, take or otherwise harm you, Muin becomes defensive and will offer a nasty sting.

Some people report this to be like a bee-sting or very painful prickle at various locations in their body. Thus Muin is the ultimate in Celtic Reiki defences!

The important thing to remember with Muin is that you never use it to hurt or harm or to create joy or balance – you just use it. The Essence will react with the energy of those you are in contact with and it is the synthesis of Muin and their intent that creates the effect. You will also find that the effects of Muin are only apparent whilst in your company, so if you use Muin and then encounter somebody who means you harm, they will only have the negative reactions to the vibrations whilst they are in your immediate space – as soon as they move to a distance where they cannot harm you, the effects will dissipate only to return if they come closer again.

Other aspects of Muin are loyalty, trust, friendship, reconciliation, abundance, prosperity, joy, happiness and the turning of the tides.

**Physical**: Diabetes and issues surrounding sugar. Also issues with challenges regarding boundaries.

**Emotional/Mental**: Loyalty amongst friends, colleagues and loved-ones. Happiness and joy, especially when seeking a blissful attitude to one's daily approach to life.

**Spiritual**: Assertion in spiritual matters. Guardianship and gatekeepers.

## *Gort – G – (Gort)*

### *The Ivy*

Gort is of the Ivy and is connected to the cerebral and psychological. The ivy creates a labyrinth – a tangle of paths and journeys. Some lead you forward, some lead you to nowhere, some lead you round and round. The Gort Essence will help you to find your way through the labyrinth, helping you to stick to the right path.

Gort can help to manifest clarity, improve memory and help you connect to higher wisdom.

He can calm the mind in times of anxiety and allow stillness in meditation. You can use Gort if you wish to manifest anonymously for the higher good, i.e., you know you need something, but you are not quite sure what.

Gort is one of the plants I have worked with extensively – from huge growths of Ivy on the side of buildings, to small potted individuals. I have harvested many varieties and this, in turn, has created a very broad energy range that can be honed down to probably the most accurate frequency of all the Celtic Essences.

Gort was the second Homoeopathic remedy created in the Celtic Tree range, created from a large plant located in Central London. It was also one of the first Celtic Vibrational Remedies, created from the vibration of Gort and a potted Ivy that I have had since she was a cutting.

**Physical**: Acts mainly on the heart for cardiac disorders. A good hangover cure!

**Emotional/Mental**: Confusion or those who feel lost. Mental haze or an overactive mind – creates stillness and focus. The Gort Essence will help you to find your way through the labyrinth, helping you to stick to the right path. Gort can help to manifest clarity, improve memory and help you connect to higher wisdom.

**Spiritual**: The main aspect of this frequency is that of spiritual enlightenment, of finding and sticking to one's path. It can free the spirit and unify energy to create a single purpose or it can branch out and raise the spirit to give a new perspective of the wider picture.

## Ngetal – Ng – (Net-tarl)

### The Broom

Ngetal is an excellent essence when dealing with excess and habitual behaviour, working on the levels of self-regulation and a deeper understanding of what is beneficial to health and what causes harm. Often associated with royalty, this plant vibration has a very 'regal' feel and is excellent for raising a person's vibration to a more expansive level, rather like Ailim, but here the emphasis is on a higher perspective of the self and one's own behaviour rather than a situation based outlook.

A general cleansing and healing 'tonic', Ngetal works on the bladder, kidneys and lymphatic system, causing detoxification through its diuretic qualities. It purges the body of substances that are harmful to health, including toxic chemicals/vibrations that the focus has been exposed to during addictive behaviour; alcohol, smoking, drugs, etc.

In the Celtic calendar, Ngetal symbolises the end of summer and the onset of the winter months, thus ushering in a time of taking stock and reconciliation. This is also seen in the Ngetal energy, as it helps a person reconcile recent events, to learn from situations and past mistakes thus enabling them to move beyond what has happened.

The cycle of sleep in order to start anew with revitalised energy reserves and a fresh, positive attitude, is also seen in Ngetal Energy as it is the vibrational equivalent of hibernation, offering the subject a chance to awaken from their treatment with newfound vigour and be completely energised. It can also create deep, restful slumber when a person is stressed or working too hard. Using Ngetal could produce a narcoleptic effect on the treatment couch and this should be noted when using it. The focus of the treatment (or Practitioner) may also find the essence nurtures them to a place where they can put down things they cling to and drop the baggage they are carrying.

The narcotic effects of Ngetal can also be used in sleep disorders – those who cannot sleep or those who are lethargic and sleep too much. The energy will help find balance and a natural, healthy routine of peaceful sleep and energised daily activity. Ngetal will help those who work shifts and have irregular sleep patterns and thus a confused 'body-clock'. Remember, however, that the energy works towards the benefit of your health and not your working objectives, so if you are dangerously over-tired, Ngetal could send you to sleep so that you get a much-needed recharge, rather than helping you to stay awake further!

The Celtic Reiki Ngetal vibration was collected from two individuals who were rescued from a discount garden centre, that was badly mistreating and neglecting their plants. The two Broom plants were near to death and crying out to passers-by in a last attempt to be saved. Once rescued, both Broom plants made a remarkable recovery and are now fully back to health, wildly energetic and have even seeded!

**Physical**: The bladder, urinary tract, kidneys, and lymphatic system. Excellent detoxifier and cleansing essence. Creates a clearing effect on the body and fluids of the body, such as blood, water, etc. Over-indulgence in food, alcohol, etc. Sleep disorders, ME and lethargy are also treated with Ngetal

**Emotional/Mental**: Taking stock of a projector period in one's life as it approaches fruition. Perhaps when one is facing a point where tough decisions need to be made about whether a project (or path) is worth continuing with. Reconciliation and consolidation.

**Spiritual**: Energy, vibrancy, power.

## *Straif – St – (Strife)*

## *The Blackthorn*

As the name suggests, the essence of Straif releases us from the trouble and strife that we encounter in our everyday lives. In many ways, Straif acts as a tonic, but it works on deeper levels than just those needed to sooth and calm – the Blackthorn vibrations extend to counteract and release all areas of darkness and pain in our lives.

Straif could be seen as a rescue remedy, as it helps those in real need; the people who can see no way out of the despair they find themselves in. It offers emergency light to what appears to be unending darkness.

Blackthorn, despite its reputation, is such a beautiful tree; the black bark and stunning blossom make it one of the most joyous celebrations of the spring, arriving before most other trees come into flower. When used in a treatment, this element of Straif can be used, for it can be placed into a treatment just before Huathe, in order to create an even deeper result when clearing the suppressed and hidden heavy energy that we spend most of our lives trying to run away from and not acknowledging as part of us.

**Physical**: Comforts the suicidal and the lost. People who self-harm or have attempted to take their life.

**Emotional/Mental**: Straif supports us in our conflicts and troubles – not just the challenges we face from time to time, but the really horrific strife that we may come across only once or twice. The Straif essence is the most wonderful essence when working with the obstacles that threaten to derail us. From hatred, vengeance, slander, libel, hate campaigns and being judged unfairly, Straif will give the strength to go on.

**Spiritual**: Straif could be seen as a rescue remedy, as it helps those in real need; the people who can see no way out of the despair they find themselves in. It offers emergency light in what appears to be unending darkness.

## Ruis – R – (Rweesh)

### The Elder

Ruis is the essence of the Elder Tree and is the perspective of birth and death, the beginning and the end. This essence allows us knowledge of the cycle of life and can be used at any time of loss and transition, including the journey beyond life. In treatments, Ruis can also be used at the beginning of any session that involves dealing with deeply embedded issues that might trigger a fear reaction or deep emotional/physical pain. When treated it will help the person to cope with these symptoms of the clearing.

In manifestation rituals, Ruis is excellent for issues surrounding the law and legal disputes. It will always work with respect for natural law, so cannot be used to sway the outcome. However, if you feel that you or your client is likely to lose the argument, it can help an amicable result to be reached thus releasing severe loss.

I received the original Essence of Ruis whilst treating an Elder in Pluckley, Kent on a hot summer's day – I can always remember the sensation of being lifted up – as if being raised to a higher place. On this occasion, something that is quite unusual for trees happened – my feet started to lift upwards, on to the toes. Usually trees are very grounding and will root the energy user to the spot, so I was intrigued by this effect.

Thus, I regularly project the Ruis Essence for those who are 'too' grounded. For example, those who focus on the physical and on material possessions or things. Ruis will lift them up to 'free' their mind and spirit and then gently ground them again, so they land in a much healthier place!

I once encountered an Elder who was dying and had roused from sleep to enjoy his last few days of life, before going on a new journey. As I held the trunk of the tree, I felt the familiar lifting sensation, although this time it was more prominent than usual. I became very aware that the tree had no fear of what was to come – he was confident of his future existence – a transcendence of death and this made me wonder if Elder could help those who are dying. Of course he can! That is his purpose – loss of life, transition and a becoming of something new and wonderful.

Soon after leaving the tree, I realised that his energy had come with me – I was carrying this tree's life force. This has remained with me ever since; for what purpose I do not yet know, however, whatever the reason I have been given this precious gift, I am confident it will be a remarkable journey!!

**Physical**: Works particularly well on sore throats or infections of the throat. The stomach is another area that would benefit from Ruis. The energy can also help with arthritis, rheumatism and sciatica.

**Emotional/Mental**: Will help the bereaved or those who have lost and need to grow before they can move on. Fear generally and especially fear of change.

**Spiritual**: Offers acceptance of one's life path, even if the person resists strongly at first – it can even create a zest for the future on a spirit's journey.

*Uilleand – Pe – Oo-lind*

*The Honeysuckle*

One thing that has always struck me about the Honeysuckle is its ability to survive through trauma and not through being strong or battling its way forward. Honeysuckle overcomes adversity through beauty, love and sweetness – the light of the Uilleand Essence reflects this and enables us to put down the 'fight' and the 'struggle', helping us to go forward and overcome our difficulties by shining with a light so bright that we can wash away darkness and shadow, working from within as opposed to fixing blame externally.

Truth comes from within us, as does fear – there is nothing outside of us that is more frightening than that which lurks within. In fact we can only be scared of things that exist within us, for, if we do not have the potential to be that thing that scares us, we cannot connect to it!

If you are afraid of the dark, it is because there is darkness within you. If you are afraid of being alone, it is because you have that loneliness within yourself and if you are frightened of being hurt, it is because you have the ability to hurt others. Uilleand enables us to see past the externalisation of our fears and helps us to look inside and shine a light to our darkest, most inaccessible parts.

This does not mean the process is a struggle or even painful, for Uilleand will help us overcome these difficulties through positive steps and healthy assertion of who we truly are. Natural command, ease of being and the conviction of walking forward with a smile are all signs of this essence and will enable the user to become much stronger than they ever thought they could be.

**Physical**: Lower abdominal issues as well as thyroid and throat dis-ease.

**Emotional/Mental**: Lethargy, depression and generally feeling 'low' are all symptoms that are eased by the application of Honeysuckle. Fizzy and vibrant, he can create laughter, the need to socialise and motivation to tackle what must be done.

**Spiritual**: Spiritual understanding and creativity . Helps us to express spiritual concepts through creation and art, as well as assisting us in understanding a spiritual ethos that is unclear, paradoxical or dogmatic.

## *Ifin – Ve – I-Vern*

## *The Fern*

Added to the Celtic Reiki System in 2006, Ifin is a welcome newcomer, as Ferns are one of the most prolific and omnipresent plants to be seen in the Celtic lands today. Decorating the hedgerows, ferns are happiness in the shade of the other trees, which protect from the harsh light of the summer sun and this is reflected in the use of Ifin Essence.

Ifin can be used wherever the brightness of healing energy creates trauma or pain – this may seem like a misnomer, yet some people are affected painfully during or after the treatment and for those who find the effects of the healing process create clearings or detoxifications that are too much to bear, Ifin will soften the affects and ease the healing process.

Ifin will also soften the 'edges' wherever you encounter a situation that is black and white, enabling the perception of the shades of grey that lay in between.

**Physical**: Burns and photosensitivity.

**Emotional/Mental**: Emotional and psychological pain and anguish. Helps those who cannot cope.

**Spiritual**: Helps alleviate the "I'm right, you're wrong" attitude, especially in spiritual circles, psychic groups, and other expanded arenas.

*Oir – Th – (U-eh)*

*The Spindle*

Oir is the Spindle, of sweetness and delight, and is used in Celtic Reiki to manifest an ideal situation. This could be more prosperity, a better job or a strengthening of relationships. Oir will help to create conducive energy for the most expansive outcome in a physical sense and therefore is best used where money, property, work or people are concerned.

Another aspect of the Spindle is that of reward. It is for those who work hard, but receive no gratitude or thanks and also for those who expect reward for everything they do. Spindle helps us carry out the tasks we must do, not for want or promise of reward, but because we should enjoy them and for the lessons we learn in the undertaking. It helps us to appreciate the journey we take rather than concentrating on the destination at the end of it.

**Physical**: Muscular pain and spasms. Issues with the left-hand-side of the body, particularly the shoulder, arm and hand. Cold sores and sores of the eyes, nose and mouth. Acne on forehead and back.

**Emotional/Mental**: Relationships, especially when attempting a reconciliation or reunion. Helps integrate knowledge and wisdom.

**Spiritual**: The learning of spiritual lessons.

## *Phagos – Ph – (Fah-gors)*

## *The Beech*

Working so extensively with Phagos has enabled the creation of not just one Beech Tree essence, but two. The vibrations of Phagos have now been split into the traditional Beech tree, and Copper Beech.

Beech is one of the most energetic trees and its vibrancy can be felt very strongly whether you are working with the youngest of saplings or the greatest of trees. The tree of wisdom and written knowledge is an interesting paradox for a race of people who did not write down their secrets, using the written word for communication and artistic purposes as opposed to wisdom.

Thus to have a tree that symbolises a concept, non-existent in its culture, offers us a new twist to the traditional Phagos Essence: to understand what cannot be and yet is. The Old Lore; a fluid verbal tradition that is older than Wicca and Druidic faiths, is never written down. Hence it is very rare and is now scarcely used, but it teaches us that when information is written down, it is fixed at that point—unchanging. It can therefore become dogma and so no longer has a place in Old Lore, which constantly changes and evolves and is added to. To remain fluid and based upon experience, as opposed to rules and 'facts', the tradition of Old Lore has to be passed down verbally from Master to Student – if ever you read any 'facts' about Old Lore, they are not Old Lore!

This is the essence of Phagos, for it symbolises written knowledge. Yet as soon as that knowledge is written, it stops being knowledge and becomes stagnant and limited. Phagos therefore provides us with the understanding of paradox and that which cannot be, for it contradicts itself. Whenever faced with a situation or subject that is a mixture of coexisting opposites and contradictions, Phagos will help us to use what cannot be to make sense of what we encounter and shift it to our understanding.

We could say that the written knowledge of Phagos is writing that we have not encountered or cannot understand yet, but exists in a way that is outside our common knowledge – like a massive encyclopaedia of energetic vibrations that we can use and interpret in our own way – this is written, but written in energy not in words. Perhaps Phagos can help us see other ways of solving the paradoxes of life?

**Physical**: Assimilation of food, excessive hunger, over-eating, eating disorders and obesity. Phagos can not only be used to help cut down on food consumption, but also to help nurture a healthy attitude towards nutrition, food and exercise.

**Emotional/Mental**: Cerebral activities, learning, reading and writing. The transmission of knowledge and expansion of the mind. Psychology and social dynamics.

**Spiritual**: The spirituality of the written word, memetics and higher beings.

## Koad or Coed – Ch – (Kode, Koy-d, or Ko-ed)

### The Grove

Koad is the essence of sacred sanctuary, of finding a place within that is calm and peaceful and will allow us to cope when everything around is falling apart. The Koad is surrounding and nurturing and protects while healing.

Koad can be used in treatment to surround and assert the client; its nature is to give peace and stillness of mind – to laugh in the face of adversity. It can also be used when other essences are not working as they should because of limiting belief or emotional patterning – it will protect the other essences from being broken down by habit and allows it to work over a period of time.

I have worked in many groves over the years, however none more so than the Rowan Grove on Bodmin Moor. This small but ancient place contains Rowan, Oak, Elder, Hazel, Gorse and many other types of tree – all of which are contained in this essence. I see the Koad Essence as a symbiotic range of vibrations – one created from many individuals, each contributing a special part of the Grove energy. There are Celtic trees here and other varieties and whilst many are already contained in the Celtic Reiki system, this conglomeration is different, as a tree reacts differently on a one to one basis than it does in a group. In Koad is the vibration of group dynamics, thus can be used on large groups of people or wherever teamwork or team spirit is needed. It can also be used to heal families.

In the vibrations of many comes a unifying dynamic that provides assertion, safety and refuge, where a person can meditate and reflect on their life, their purpose and their mission. Koad is an essence that envelops, and in which you can lose yourself for a while.

**Physical:** Koad works wonders on the nervous system and can have an effect on everything from mild-stress to major nervous disorders. It can be used for Raynaud's Syndrome, numbness, paralysis or palsy. It can also work with hyperactivity, or lethargy, and anywhere where there is too much or too little of something (hyper/hypoglycaemia, hypo/hypertension, etc.)

**Emotional/Mental:** An overactive mind or imagination. Too much internal monologue – no peace and quite. Helps a person to remain calm and still even when all around them is falling apart. Introspection (lack of or too much of)

**Spiritual:** A spiritual sanctuary, a place of being in the moment.

# Acknowledgements

To my tree friends and those who have contributed to the Celtic Reiki system; everyone who has helped me on these adventures and the Celtic Reiki Masters who have given their most precious commodity (time) and effort to preserving the oral traditions and the integrity of the practice. For those who cherish Celtic Reiki and see the precious nature of this gift we have been given.

To my students and those who have walked by my side in all kinds of weather. We have tippy-toed through the most fantastic and beautiful memories; moments that are so profound we become tearful when we remember them; laughter to the extent of severe pain; and a few dark times too. Your kindness, support, and words of encouragement are a total inspiration to me. Thank you.

To my parents. For getting me here and for being there. For learning with me and for journeying through all we have been through. For all the laughs and for every occasion we have managed to clear a restaurant! To my brothers who are just the most fun on six legs. Now why didn't I think of that years ago!!?

To all my friends – I don't need a reason, you're all just wonderful, beautiful people!!

Thank you to Richard for being an inspiration!

And gratitude goes out to those who have given me the opportunity to grow strong and to become wiser.

**The Celtic Reiki Home Experience**

If you would like to experience the wonder of Celtic Reiki Mastership with Martyn Pentecost, you can discover the rich and immersive adventure of the mPowr Celtic Reiki Home Experience -

http://www.mpowrunlimited.com.

*Also by Martyn Pentecost & published by mPowr:*

***The Official Guide to Celtic Reiki:***
***A Walk in the Forest***
ISBN: 978-1907282003

***Celtic Reiki Mastery: A Workbook***
ISBN: 978-1907282027

***Karmic Regression Therapy & Karmic Reiki:***
***An Official Guide***
ISBN: 978-1907282034

***vPsychic***
ISBN: 978-1907282041

**Available in 2010**

***vPsychic Adventures***
ISBN: 978-1907282058

***Beyond vPsychic: The iLayer Phenomena***
ISBN: 978-1907282065